MW01620921

The Political Life of an Epidemic

Zimbabwe's catastrophic cholera outbreak of 2008–09 saw an unprecedented number of people affected, with 100,000 cases and nearly 5,000 deaths. Cholera, however, was much more than a public health crisis: it represented the nadir of the country's deepening political and economic crisis of 2008.

This study focuses on the political life of the cholera epidemic, tracing the historical origins of the outbreak, examining the social pattern of its unfolding and impact, analysing the institutional and communal responses to the disease, and marking the effects of its aftermath.

Across different social and institutional settings, competing interpretations and experiences of the cholera epidemic created charged social and political debates. In his examination of these debates which surrounded the breakdown of Zimbabwe's public health infrastructure and failing bureaucratic order, the scope and limitations of disaster relief, and the country's profound levels of livelihood poverty and social inequality, Simukai Chigudu reveals how this epidemic of a preventable disease had profound implications for political institutions and citizenship in Zimbabwe.

SIMUKAI CHIGUDU is Associate Professor of African Politics at the University of Oxford and Fellow of St Antony's College, Oxford. He was awarded the biennial Audrey Richards Prize for the best doctoral thesis in African Studies examined at a UK university. He is the author of several articles in leading academic journals including *African Affairs*, *Critical African Studies*, and *Health Policy and Planning*. He worked as a medical doctor before moving into academia.

The Political Life of an Epidemic

Cholera, Crisis and Citizenship in Zimbabwe

SIMUKAI CHIGUDU
University of Oxford

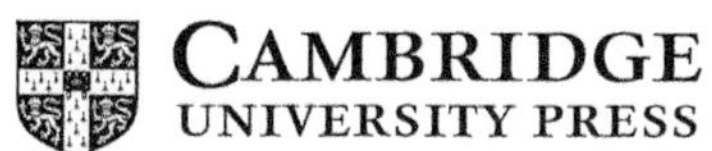

CAMBRIDGE
UNIVERSITY PRESS

University Printing House, Cambridge CB2 8BS, United Kingdom

One Liberty Plaza, 20th Floor, New York, NY 10006, USA

477 Williamstown Road, Port Melbourne, VIC 3207, Australia

314–321, 3rd Floor, Plot 3, Splendor Forum, Jasola District Centre, New Delhi – 110025, India

79 Anson Road, #06–04/06, Singapore 079906

Cambridge University Press is part of the University of Cambridge.

It furthers the University's mission by disseminating knowledge in the pursuit of education, learning, and research at the highest international levels of excellence.

www.cambridge.org
Information on this title: www.cambridge.org/9781108489102
DOI: 10.1017/9781108773928

First published 2020

Printed in the United Kingdom by TJ International Ltd, Padstow Cornwal

A catalogue record for this publication is available from the British Library.

Library of Congress Cataloging-in-Publication Data
Names: Chigudu, Simukai, 1986– author.
Title: The political life of an epidemic : cholera, crisis and citizenship in Zimbabwe / Simukai Chigudu.
Description: New York : Cambridge University Press, 2020. | Includes bibliographical references and index.
Identifiers: LCCN 2019042513 (print) | LCCN 2019042514 (ebook) | ISBN 9781108489102 (hardback) | ISBN 9781108733441 (paperback) | ISBN 9781108773928 (epub)
Subjects: LCSH: Cholera–Zimbabwe. | Cholera–Political aspects–Zimbabwe. | Cholera–Social aspects–Zimbabwe. | Public health–Zimbabwe. | Public health administration–Zimbabwe.
Classification: LCC RA644.C3 C45 2020 (print) | LCC RA644.C3 (ebook) | DDC 362.1969320096891–dc23
LC record available at https://lccn.loc.gov/2019042513
LC ebook record available at https://lccn.loc.gov/2019042514

ISBN 978-1-108-48910-2 Hardback

For Hope and Tafi
&
For Mr J, we made it.

Contents

Figures

Table

Preface

I was in my fifth year of medical school at Newcastle University when I first stumbled upon a startling article in *The New York Times* entitled, 'Cholera Epidemic Sweeping across Crumbling Zimbabwe' (Dugger 2008). The piece, published in early December 2008, began by recounting how the disease had claimed the lives of the five youngest members of the Chigudu family with 'cruel and bewildering haste'. The children had been playing in the sewage-flooded streets of a Harare township, gleefully unaware of the deadly bacteria lurking therein. It was only a matter of hours before all five children began purging and vomiting. Within less than a day, they were limp and hollow-eyed as life seeped out of their desiccated bodies. 'Then they started to die', said their brother Lovegot, 'Prisca was first, second Sammy, then Shantel, Clopas and Aisha, the littlest one, last' (Dugger 2008). *The New York Times*, along with numerous other media agencies as well as regional and international organisations, reported that this outbreak was indisputable evidence that Zimbabwe's most fundamental public services – including water and sanitation, public schools and hospitals – had shut down, much like the organs of a severely dehydrated cholera victim. The spread and lethality of the disease did not abate. The country's public health systems floundered in response to a straightforward bacterial infection – one that is easy to prevent, difficult to spread, and simple to treat. Over the course of ten months, Zimbabwe's cholera outbreak reached catastrophic proportions that are almost unrivalled in the modern history of the disease.

Throughout 2008, I felt like I was drowning, engulfed by a deluge of disaster reports, articles, opinion pieces, blogs and analyses of the situation in Zimbabwe. From rigged elections to political violence, a desperate economy and the collapse of public services, cholera was now the latest in a litany of catastrophes.

I could not afford the ticket home that December. Even if I could, I would be impotent to help. It terrified me that four and a half years of medical school in the United Kingdom could not prepare me to work in such conditions: Zimbabwe's major hospitals, including the renowned Parirenyatwa General Hospital, had effectively shut down, the health system largely reduced to ad hoc cholera camps where forlorn and heroic medical students, doctors, nurses and other volunteers worked tirelessly to pump fluids into the collapsed veins of ailing bodies. Those patients were the lucky ones. The majority of cholera's victims did not reach the camps, left at home instead to defaecate violently while courting death.

News outlets from across the world seized upon this opportunity to remind us that Zimbabwe, 'a pariah state', was left in tatters owing to the whims of an ageing and despotic leader. Accusations and counter-accusations proliferated. Surely, argued much Western intelligentsia, cholera was irrefutable proof that Zimbabwe was a failed state – after all, only the most callous and self-interested of political leaders could preside over a health crisis of this magnitude. Zimbabwean officials hit back with equal fervour and belligerence, the now late Minister of Information notoriously decrying cholera as racist, terrorist, biological warfare from the West to undermine African sovereignty.

For a time, global health activists at my medical school insisted that we must 'do something' about the cholera outbreak. Deep down, I suspected that the alacrity would not last. How could it be otherwise? Darfur, Somalia, Palestine and the Congo were all competing for our compassion, our attention, our naive idealism.

I always knew the situation was more complicated and more important than 800-word op-eds would lead me to think. Why had the country's water systems failed so badly? Why was poor Budiriro so remorselessly afflicted while wealthy Borrowdale only heard rumours of diarrhoea? What did cholera have to tell us about public policy, about disputes over the social distribution of power, status and economic rewards in Zimbabwe? How were people surviving? What did it mean to live through such wanton suffering?

Many years passed, cholera all but forgotten. I continued with my clinical training, passed my exams and began a life of ward rounds, on-calls, and night shifts in the United Kingdom's slowly privatising National Health Service. I had hoped that clinical practice would give me direction and purpose that I could channel back towards home one day. The experience of watching cholera at a distance remained emblematic of my sense of dislocation. It accentuated the chasm

I saw between my professional training and socialisation in the United Kingdom and events in Zimbabwe. I carried with me deep feelings of longing, isolation and responsibility.

Medicine was always both comfortable and unsettling for me. Self-consciously expert-based, technology-driven, financially secure and benevolent, the profession easily justifies itself as a sensible career choice. The daily routine of treating the sick is undoubtedly rewarding but leaves little room to look beyond individual pathology and consider questions of context, of power and of structural violence in shaping patterns of disease and experiences of illness. I eventually left medicine to make a new start as an academic in the social sciences, to reconnect with my home country's fraught politics while protected by analytical distance.

This book, the final product of my doctoral studies, realises my conversion from medical doctor to social scientist. It is therefore a very personal project but one that has come into being through the considerable guidance, wisdom and support from numerous teachers, colleagues and friends over several years. Among them, few deserve more credit than my doctoral supervisor.

From the moment I had my first thoughts about studying the politics of cholera to the very final stages of drafting this book, Professor Jocelyn Alexander has been a unique source of encouragement. At each stage of my reading, writing and research, Joss has pushed me to think rigorously and broadly, to take ownership of my project, to craft a distinct scholarly identity, and to argue with conviction and passion about my subject matter. I cannot express how much I have learnt from Joss or how much I have matured as a thinker under her supervision.

I have been extremely lucky to receive further mentorship and intellectual guidance from Jonny Steinberg, whose unmatched creativity has encouraged me to see new ideas and possibilities in my own work. Similarly, Miles Tendi, Megan Vaughan, Tom Scott-Smith and Sloan Mahone have all read my work at various stages, and their input permeates this book in a multitude of ways. At Cambridge University Press, Maria Marsh has been a fantastic advocate of my work, while the two anonymous reviewers of the book made powerful suggestions to enhance the quality of my writing and argumentation.

This book would not have been possible without the funding that supported my doctoral studies during which time the bulk of the research was carried out. I am grateful for the generosity of the Weidenfeld-Hoffman Trust whose scholarship programme allowed me to study at Oxford, and I am thankful for the additional support provided to me by St Anne's College, Oxford.

Words cannot do justice to my gratitude to all those who participated in this study. I am especially appreciative of the time and diligence of Winnet Shamuyarira who organised most of my focus group discussions and whose well-earned street credibility gave me access to people and communities far outside of my own circles. Amos Matembe and Favor Makovore kindly spent hours on end accompanying me around Harare's high-density townships, often acting as a mediators and interpreters through many of my interviews.

My academic community in Oxford has had a transformative impact on me. I am thankful to friends and colleagues at the Oxford Department of International Development. It has been a pleasure to be part of the teaching staff in the department and to see how world-class scholars approach research and pedagogy. Similarly, the African Studies Centre has been a second intellectual home, and its faculty, affiliated lecturers and administrative staff have supported me in innumerable ways. Over the years, I have learnt a great deal from Neil Carrier, Nic Cheeseman, Cheryl Doss, Doug Gollin, Miles Larmer, Olly Owen, David Pratten, Andrea Purdekova and Ricardo Soares de Oliveira. Beyond Oxford, I am thankful for the support and engagement of Julie Balen and David McCoy.

I am indebted to the administrative and support staff at ODID who have made my life easy by allowing me to conduct my academic work with minimal bureaucratic hassle. And I'm equally indebted to my students who have challenged and inspired me with their curiosity, convictions and thirst for knowledge.

There are so many friends who have spurred me on and brought me more joy and comfort than they could possibly imagine. I cannot name them all here but I must give special acknowledgement to Tom Burgoine, Mihika Chatterjee, Arnold Chamunogwa, Michaela Collord, Natalya Din-Kariuki, Kieran Gilfoy, Mona Hakimi, Max Harris, Dan Hodgkinson, Sa'eed Husaini, Hayley Jones, Yasmin Kumi, Zaad Mahmood, Kuukuwa Manful, Ankita Pandey, Joe Piper, James Smith, Sanjeev Srirathan, Harry Verhoeven, Chris Wilkinson, Martin Williams and Arturo Zoffman-Rodríguez.

Barry Knight, Christine Morrison and James Morrison-Knight have been a second family to me since I moved to England. Back home, I am thankful to the late Mr J, who gave so much of himself to ensure my happiness, as well as to Kuda and Rudo Chigudu who are constant companions and inspirations.

Tafi and Hope Chigudu: you have taught me, throughout my life's journey, to believe in myself far beyond any latent potential I have previously shown. Through this you have unlocked my imagination and raised me to be the man that I am: always free to follow my own dreams and chart my own way through life. I love you and I thank you. I dedicate this book to you.

Finally, a note about the stories I tell in this book.

I must acknowledge at the outset that the retelling of cholera narratives plays a crucial part in shaping their social and political impact. Each of my interlocutors spoke to me with warmth and openness, kindness and patience, even as I insisted on asking awkward and painful questions about politics, disease, suffering and death. I am grateful for the vulnerability with which my interlocutors shared their stories of the cholera outbreak. I cannot possibly hope to bring out the full texture of the complex narratives I was told. Inevitably, I have forged my own analysis by extracting stories from the words of my interlocutors and by selectively reading the settings in which their words emerge. I take all responsibility for any distortions and misrepresentations in this text while I also aim, throughout the book, to be as transparent as possible about my intellectual choices and the limitations of my observations.

With this acknowledgement comes a sharp awareness of the ethical baggage that a book of this nature carries. Foremost among my ethical concerns is a dilemma encapsulated in a question from a teenage girl, Chido, in the high-density suburb of Glen Norah. A gregarious presence and candid interviewee, Chido's narration of the outbreak was poignant and affecting. At the end of our discussion, she pointedly asked me, 'Are you going to help us?' My response was sheepish, even if true, 'I'm going to try but there is nothing much that I can do. The way I can help is very indirect. There are many of us who are trying to write about what was happening in 2008. We want to use our writing to influence the way things need to change.' I doubt I convinced her. I suspect Chido welcomed my presence and intrusive questions only as mild reprieve from an otherwise mundane afternoon. It is perhaps after encounters such as these that I most acutely miss the tangible results, the direct engagement, the measurable progress and the visible satisfaction that clinical medicine can provide. Is my book then mere pontification? A self-indulgent and extractive, even exploitative, immersion into other people's suffering?

Charles Briggs (2004: 16) motivated his study of a cholera outbreak in the Orinocco Delta of Venezuela by saying, 'I feel it is particularly important to convey this information to as wide an audience as possible because much of it has been actively suppressed, thereby precluding more visible and substantive responses on the part of national and international audiences and organizations.' The physician-anthropologist, Didier Fassin (2007b: xxii–xxiii), begins his monograph on the experience and politics of AIDS in South Africa fully confident of the social value of his work:

> [M]y political view of anthropology is also a moral one. I believe the work presented here can be socially useful, that anthropology is not a matter of art for art's sake, that making the things of this world a bit more intelligible, especially when they appear opaque, and irrational, can make them less unjust, ineluctable, or unacceptable. To put it bluntly (of course, in a Durkheimian tradition), I am convinced that social science would not be worth a moment's attention or labour if it had no political role.

I would like to think that this book is important for more than its contribution to academe, for more than the advancement of my career, and for more than my personal edification. What comes to mind – not for the last time in this work – is a passage from Albert Camus's classic humanist novel, *The Plague*, about an awful outbreak that gripped the coastal city of Oran in Algeria. At the end of the novel, the narrator, revealed to be the protagonist Dr Rieux, explains his compulsion to compile his chronicle, 'so that he should not be one of those who hold their peace but should bear witness in favor of those plague-stricken people; so that some memorial of the injustices and outrage done them might endure' (Camus 1967: 251). May this book also serve as a memorial of the injustice and outrage done to those whose lives were devastated by Zimbabwe's cholera outbreak.

Abbreviations

C4	Cholera Command and Control Centre
CBD	Central Business District
CDC	Centers for Disease Control and Prevention
CHRA	Combined Harare Residents' Association
CIO	Central Intelligence Organisation
CMA	Critical Medical Anthropology
DRC	Democratic Republic of the Congo
GNU	Government of National Unity
GOARN	Global Outbreak Alert and Response Network
GOZ	Government of Zimbabwe
HIV/AIDS	Human Immunodeficiency Virus/Acquired Immunodeficiency Syndrome
ICDDR-B	International Centre for Diarrhoeal Disease Research, Bangladesh
ICG	International Crisis Group
ICRC	International Committee of the Red Cross
IOM	International Organization for Migration
IRC	International Rescue Committee
MDC	Movement for Democratic Change
MDC-M	Movement for Democratic Change–Mutambara
MDC-T	Movement for Democratic Change–Tsvangirai
MoHCW	Ministry of Health and Child Welfare
MSF	Médecins Sans Frontières
NGOs	Non-Governmental Organisations
ORT	Oral Rehydration Therapy
PHR	Physicians for Human Rights
PVO	Private Voluntary Organisations
UANC	United African National Council
UN	United Nations

UNICEF	United Nations Children's Fund
UNOCHA	United Nations Office for the Coordination of Humanitarian Affairs
WHO	World Health Organization
ZADHR	Zimbabwe Association of Doctors for Human Rights
ZANLA	Zimbabwe National Liberation Army
ZANU(PF)	Zimbabwe African National Union, Patriotic Front
ZAPU	Zimbabwe African People's Union
ZINWA	Zimbabwe National Water Authority
ZIPRA	Zimbabwe People's Revolutionary Army
ZLHR	Zimbabwe Lawyers for Human Rights
ZNA	Zimbabwe National Army
ZWD	Zimbabwe Dollar

Map of Zimbabwe

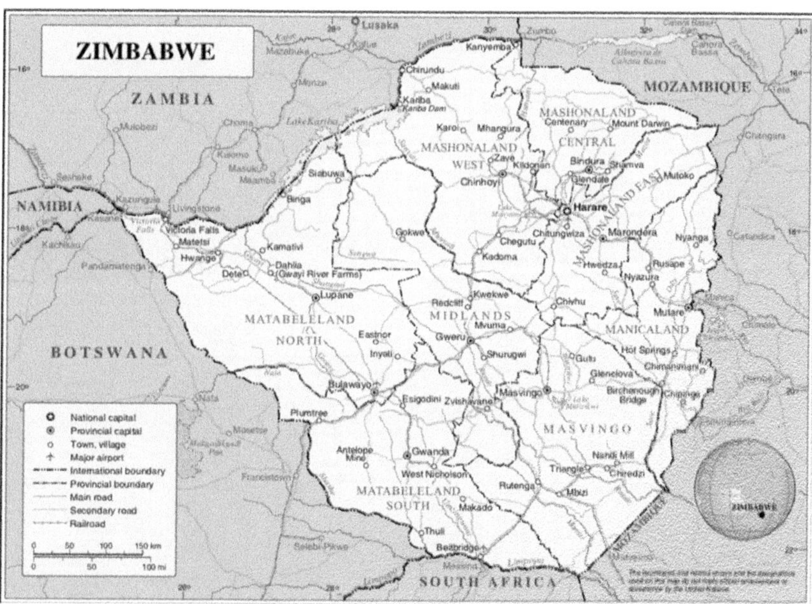

Source: UN Cartographic Section

Introduction

Stories and Politics of Cholera

I am bored, but there is a great deal that is interesting in cholera if you look at it from a detached point of view.

—Anton Chekhov, *Letters of Anton Chekhov*, 1892

In August 2008, the impoverished high-density townships of Harare's metropolitan area were engulfed by a devastating cholera outbreak. The epidemic quickly spread into peri-urban and rural areas in Zimbabwe before crossing the country's borders into South Africa, Botswana, Zambia and Mozambique. Over the course of ten months, the disease infected over 98,000 people and claimed over 4,000 lives; with an exceptionally high case-fatality rate at the peak of the epidemic, Zimbabwe's 2008 cholera outbreak has been deemed the largest and most extensive in recorded African history (Mason 2009). Epidemiologically, the outbreak can be explained by the breakdown and cross-contamination of the city's water and sanitation systems. Such a reading, however, belies the complex interaction of political, economic and historical factors that initially gave rise to the dysfunction of the water systems, that delineate the socio-spatial pattern of the outbreak, and that account for the fragmented and inadequate response of the national health system (Musemwa 2010). Cholera then was not only a public health crisis; it also signalled new dimension to the country's deepening political and economic crisis in 2008, which brought into question the capacity and legitimacy of the state.

In this book, I am not seeking to address the cholera outbreak as a technical problem to be solved or to be prevented in future. Indeed there already exists a rich epidemiological literature speaking to this very question (see, for example, Neseni and Guzha 2009; Stephenson 2009; Hove-Musekwa et al. 2011; Luque Fernández et al. 2011; Mukandavire et al. 2011; Luque Fernandez et al. 2012). Instead, this book is about the political life of the cholera epidemic. It examines the epidemic's origins, the pattern of its unfolding, its social impact, official and communal responses to it, and its aftermath in civic and public life. Across different institutional settings, competing interpretations and experiences of cholera created a series of charged social and political debates about the breakdown of Zimbabwe's public health infrastructure and failing bureaucratic order, about the scope and limits of national and international agencies in the delivery of disaster relief, and about the country's profound levels of livelihood poverty and social inequality. Examining the political life of this epidemic offers compelling insights into politics, humanitarianism, social inequality, the state and citizenship in Africa.

This book sets out to answer three principal questions. *First, what were the historical and political-economic factors that account for the origins and scale of the cholera outbreak?* Through this question, I explore how the cholera outbreak maps onto a dense and complex political history of the establishment, transformation and disruption of urban order in Harare. Such an analysis sheds new light on changes in Zimbabwe's bureaucracy, on its contentious urban politics, and on the co-constitutive entanglement of the material environment (such as Harare's hydraulic infrastructure) with social arrangements (such as how people live in, manage and negotiate urban spaces). *Second, how did different organisational entities, communities and individuals act in response to the cholera outbreak?* Through this question, I explore how one disease, cholera, gave rise to many different crises thereby engendering multiple, often competing experiences of the outbreak as well as multiple, often competing modes of addressing it. In effect, cholera took on a variety of forms depending on where and by whom it was encountered. Cholera's fraught politics emerge from the multiple crises it engendered and from its embeddedness in extant political conflicts and social relations. *Third, how has the cholera outbreak been committed to historical memory and what political subjectivities has the epidemic generated?* Through this question, I explore the myriad memories and meanings that cholera has left in civic and public life. I uncover these meanings from the stories people tell about the outbreak. I consider why these narratives take the forms that they do. And I examine what political subjectivities these stories reveal after such a marked period of social suffering.

Cholera as an indicator and a test of social and political systems has occupied a central place in much of the non-medical literature on the subject, and it provides a guiding thread that runs through this book.

The historian Richard Evans (2006: 474), in his ground-breaking history of cholera in Hamburg in the latter part of the nineteenth century, advocates the study of the disease in this manner but rightfully cautions that 'we need to be very careful and circumspect in handling this way of approaching cholera.' In Evans's survey of the literature on the great cholera outbreaks of Europe's industrial revolution, he notes a tendency among historians to ascribe to cholera the power to bring about 'social breakdown' or to reinforce 'social stability'. He notes, for instance, historical accounts of the 1832 cholera outbreak in Britain, in which it is argued that cholera did not usher in 'social breakdown', but instead acted as 'a stimulus to a whole range of sanitary reforms, to a series of transformations in the administration of public health, to the initiation of major schemes of slum clearance, and to long-term improvements in housing and living conditions' (Evans 2006: 473). While expressing admiration for such studies, Evans critiques the analytical imprecision with which terms such as social stability or its breakdown are invoked. Moreover, he argues, 'it takes a lot more than an epidemic to cause the destruction of a political and social system' (Evans 2006: 474) or, for that matter, to radically transform it. Social transformation, stability or breakdown are always a matter of politics.

For Evans, the cholera outbreaks that plagued social and political life in Hamburg in the late nineteenth and early twentieth centuries are best understood as 'events that ... might perhaps be ultimately insignificant in themselves, but nevertheless, as in a flash of lightning, illuminate a whole historical landscape' (Evans 2006: 567). As he elegantly articulates it, during a cholera outbreak, 'the workings of state and society, the structures of social inequality, the variety of values and beliefs, the physical contours of everyday life, the formal ideologies and informal ambitions of political organisations' (Evans 2006: ix) are all thrown into sharp and detailed relief. The study of cholera, therefore, reveals a great deal about a society through the factors that led to its emergence, through its unfolding and through its consequences. I approach this study of Zimbabwe's 2008–09 cholera outbreak along similar lines: as an event that might ultimately be insignificant in itself but one which opens a window unto many aspects of the country's historical, social and political landscapes that are otherwise left obscure.

Over the coming pages, I travel with cholera through time and space to illuminate the urban history of Harare and the structural factors that have left high-density residential areas prone to diarrhoeal disease outbreaks; to show that the political disruptions wrought by Zimbabwe's post-2000 crisis had unforeseen and catastrophic consequences for human health; to reveal the inherently pluralistic nature of an epidemic and the divisive politics that accompany it; and to make apparent how a medical nightmare marks the social contours of life and death, belonging and exclusion, privilege and abjection within the body politic.

Situating the Book

A study conceived along the lines described above necessarily cuts across conventional disciplinary boundaries. This project is emphatically not a specialist work of public health or social epidemiology. I approach a public health event from the point of view of an interdisciplinary social scientist rather than a health scientist. My thinking has been informed by work in the disciplines of politics, history, sociology and anthropology. My goal is to link the structural (politics, economics, history) to the subjective (experiences, memories, imagination) through the prism of cholera. In the following subsections I discuss the literatures I draw upon to make this analytical move.

Political Order and the Bureaucratic State

Throughout the annals of African political history, scholars from wide-ranging intellectual traditions and theoretical inclinations have grappled with how best to conceptualise the African state, its political and economic trajectory, and its relationship to wider society. Political scientists and political economists, in particular, have been preoccupied with one fundamental question in this analytical task: Why have African states 'proved to be such weak *Leviathans* or, phrased in more normative terms, why they have failed to generate meaningful public goods?' (Nugent 2010: 38).

Prominent writings about African politics from the 1980s to the present day have posited various historical and structural factors as having explanatory power for the nature of states across the continent. Concepts such as 'extraversion' (Bayart 2000), 'gatekeeping' (Cooper 2002), an inability to 'broadcast power' (Herbst 2000), the role of geography in shaping state formation and the distribution of power

(Clapham 2017), 'weak capacity' (Englebert and Tull 2008) and so forth have been invoked by analysts to suggest that African states are inherently weak and contradictory in nature: strong at the centre but powerless in the periphery, ambitious in aspiration but feeble in service provision, nationalist in rhetoric but divisive in reality, patrimonial in orientation but modern in institutional context (see also Bayart 1986; Chabal 1986; Geschiere 1988; Migdal 1988). Moreover, the violence and illiberal politics characterising large swathes of the continent, most starkly manifested in the breakdown of order in countries like Somalia, Sierra Leone and Zaire/Democratic Republic of the Congo in the 1990s, popularised a 'failed state' narrative in Africa. In this perspective, African states are understood not in terms of what they are, but what they have failed to be (W. Jones, Soares de Oliveira and Verhoeven 2013). Relatedly, a sophisticated literature on the 'shadow state' (for example, Reno 1999) has advanced the analysis of the political economy of war-torn states and provided nuanced accounts of their workings, but most of these notable studies focused on 'warlords' with often inchoate ideas of the state, short-term planning horizons and personal rule operating without bureaucratic institutions. Such trends may have been representative of countries like wartime Liberia. However, they could not be generalised to African state trajectories as a whole (Hagmann and Péclard 2010).

Another important explanatory paradigm of the African state is that of 'neo-patrimonialism' (Bratton and Van De Walle 1994). Deploying the metaphor of the African state as a ship that does not seek to go anywhere but rather stay afloat (R. H. Jackson and Rosberg 1982), proponents of this perspective highlight 'neo-patrimonial management strategies of elites and the attempted stabilisation of the polity through temporary alliances, ethnic coalition-building and the cynical manipulation of electoral systems and federalism' (W. Jones, Soares de Oliveira and Verhoeven 2013). Ruling elites are thus untroubled by persisting state weakness and seek neither lasting transformation of society nor fundamental change of Africa's marginalisation in the international system. The political instrumentalisation of dysfunctionality to retain power is embodied in figures like Mobutu Sese Seko, Daniel arap Moi and Blaise Compaoré. As Patrick Chabal and Jean-Pascal Daloz (1999: 15–16) put it in their seminal work,

> [T]he notion that [African] politicians, bureaucrats or military chiefs should be the servants of the state does not make sense. Their political obligations are, first and foremost, to their kith and kin, their clients, their communities, their regions, or even to their religion. All such patrons seek ideally to constitute themselves as 'Big Men', controlling as many networks as they can ... We are thus led to conclude that, in most African countries, the state is no more than a décor, a pseudo-Western façade masking the realities of deeply personalized political realities.

Thus much work in political science has come to portray African states in virtually pathological categories (Hagmann and Péclard 2010). The proliferation of terms such as 'weakness' (R. H. Jackson and Rosberg 1982), 'fragility' (Stewart and Brown 2009), 'failure' (Rotberg 2002) and 'collapse' (Zartman 1995) when describing Africa's states attests to this. We are left with a nightmarish image of 'shadow' (Reno 1999) or 'quasi' (Hopkins 2000) states that lack both popular legitimacy and administrative capacity. However, very little in this literature give us much of an understanding of the state and its institutions as such. Instead, two dominant modes of analysis prevail in which the African state is defined with negative reference to some normative, but often unspecified, conception of the good or else is dismissed as an elaborate fiction where personal networks of power matter much more for politics than do actual institutions.

The pre-eminence of the 'failed states' and neo-patrimonialism paradigms in the study of the state and politics in Africa has been challenged increasingly by numerous scholars in the disciplines of politics, history and anthropology. These literatures tend to support the view that bureaucratic institutions, historical legacies and ideologies of service provision are important (Nugent 2010).

For instance, the 'political settlements' literature – emerging out of Mushtaq Khan's (1995) work in the mid-1990s – differs from the neo-patrimonialism literature on clientelism. The main problem with the neo-patrimonial school, from a political settlements perspective, is that it provides a limited account of how clientelist political practices vary across the continent or across time and how forms of such politics interact with other forms of political mobilisation. This literature places emphasis on examining the debates, links and rival interests within and between different arms of the state; understanding the challenges of governing political coalitions; and considering how the state's links to non-state actors, in the private sector or in development organisations, influences various aspects of political praxis (Behuria, Buur and Gray 2017).

Similarly, since the late 1990s, there has been a burgeoning of scholarship on contemporary statehood that can collectively be termed 'anthropology of the state' (see Hansen and Stepputat 2001; Das and Poole 2004; Blundo and Sardan 2006; Sharma and Gupta 2006; Blundo and Meur 2009). An anthropological interrogation of the state, Aradhana Sharma and Akhil Gupta (2006) argue, is one that examines representations of the state as well as its everyday activities. Anthropologists of the state assume a plurality of power centres within, adjacent to and partially intertwined with the state (Bierschenk and Olivier de Sardan 2014). However, they make the crucial point that within such a complex field of power, states remain powerful sites of symbolic and cultural production that use metaphors and imagery to help 'secure their legitimacy, to naturalize their authority, and to represent themselves as superior to, and encompassing of, other institutions and centers of power' (Ferguson and Gupta 2002: 982).

Representations of the state are especially important at times of crisis when the legitimacy of the government is being contested hence, for instance, the morally and politically charged public discourse during the cholera epidemic, which I will highlight at many points through the book. In the realm of practice, anthropologists insightfully point out that 'state processes' are fragmentary and often carried out through a variegated apparatus of state and non-state institutions and actors. Thomas Bierschenck and Jean-Pierre Olivier de Sardan advocate for an anthropology that deals with state institutions on this basis. This approach, they assert, should not focus on a bounded research object – 'the state' as a clearly definable unit of analysis – but 'on ethnographic investigations of the properties of the phenomena, processes and practices connected to state institutions, state authority and the state provision of services and good, that is their "stateness" or state quality' (Bierschenk and Olivier de Sardan 2014: 15).

The pivotal message, therefore, is that institutions in Africa are neither elaborate fictions nor a cover for something else, but help to inform the behaviour of official and non-state actors alike in fundamental ways (Nugent 2010). Put another way, the state is a specific, historically constituted way of organising a universe of communities: it is simultaneously an instrument for accumulation and the management of rents, an important battleground for elite conflict, and a constellation of diverse institutions often contending with everyday realities, such as the scarcity of human resources and logistics and the inadequacy of official remuneration (see Verhoeven 2015: 25–29).

When analysing the history and character of the Zimbabwean state to help explain the politics of the cholera outbreak, I eschew the categories of 'state failure' and neo-patrimonialism. While elements of both these conceptions of the African state may be present in the Zimbabwean case, important experiences are not captured. Instead I draw inspiration from work that pays serious attention to the formation and trajectory of the country's strong bureaucracies and how these have been used to craft political order. As Jocelyn Alexander and JoAnn McGregor (2013: 749) explain, Zimbabwe's powerful state bureaucracies, its liberation struggle history, its substantial formal sector and its strong post-independence history of service provision had all seemed to mark it out as different from the experience of those Central and West African countries that had often provided the empirical basis for theories of state 'failure' and social and political disorder. Assumptions that African states were 'weak' or ideas about neo-patrimonial rule have frequently left no space for the narrative and ideological weight of liberation struggle legacies or the inheritance of centralised bureaucratic states.

I argue that the Zimbabwean state is best understood historically as bureaucratic and powerful. In this way, the political disruptions of the late 1990s onwards – and indeed the cholera outbreak of 2008–09 – are all the more striking and require careful, contextual scrutiny. I turn to a discussion about the trajectory of the Zimbabwean state now to flesh out the shifting dynamics of bureaucracy and political order in the country.

During Zimbabwe's transition to independence and black majority rule in 1980, the incoming government inherited a highly technocratic, centralised and powerful bureaucratic state apparatus from its Rhodesian predecessor. The new ruling party, the Zimbabwe African National Union Patriotic Front (ZANU(PF)), was quick to put this powerful machine to use in the service of 'modernising development' (Alexander 2010). Throughout the 1980s, the majority of Zimbabweans gained unprecedented access to education and health care, while a large land resettlement programme for the benefit of rural people was underway. Of note, the government made remarkable progress in the provision of water and sanitation to rural households, winning praise from the World Health Organization (WHO) and UNICEF for its ability to provide safe drinking water to 84 per cent of the national population by 1988 (Muzondidya 2009). By the 1990s, Zimbabwe could proudly claim a substantial middle class, an educated population, a diversified economy and a sophisticated infrastructure. Crucially, Alexander (2010) notes, the ZANU(PF) government derived legitimacy as a result of its capacity to deliver development.

In 2008, however, the situation could scarcely look any more different. After a decade-long economic slide, annual inflation rates – somewhere in the region of 231 million per cent according to official statistics (Reserve Bank of Zimbabwe 2008) and estimated by independent economists at 89.7 sextillion per cent (Hanke and Kwok 2009) – had reached world record–setting levels. Public services, including health and education, had largely disintegrated. Major shortages of basic commodities had been piled on top of political turmoil and violence. And cholera was competing for lives with one of the highest HIV rates in the world (Hammar, Raftopoulos and Jensen 2003; Lopman et al. 2006; Bond 2007; Raftopoulos 2009; Muzondidya 2009). The 1990s are often cited as epochal in Zimbabwe's transition from 'modernising development' to 'crisis'. This period saw a shift in the social and political forces in the country during which the popular legitimacy of the ruling party declined while concurrently a range of social movements cohered into the most successful opposition party in post-colonial Zimbabwe, the Movement for Democratic Change (MDC), formed in 1999. The MDC presented ZANU(PF) with its first real possibility of electoral defeat in the general and presidential elections in 2000 and 2002, respectively (Raftopoulos 2009). From 2000 onwards, an upheaval – widely referred to as 'the crisis' – consisting of a combination of economic decline, authoritarian nationalism and violence came to define Zimbabwe's changing political landscape.

There are a multitude of accounts regarding the origins of the crisis. Here I highlight two major but contrasting lines of argument: the first examines continuities and ruptures in Zimbabwe's internal politics to explain the crisis; the second lends more weight to ZANU(PF)'s embeddedness in and revolt against an exploitative and neo-imperialist global economy in its explanation. These two frames shape much of the popular discourse about politics in Zimbabwe, as will become clearer later in the book when I examine the disputatious polemics around cholera in detail (see Chapter 3).

In the first frame, several authors argue that when faced with declining popular legitimacy and a major political threat in the form of the MDC, ZANU(PF) drew on a discourse of revived nationalism – organised around a particular, 'patriotic' reading of the country's history (Ranger 2004; Tendi 2010) – that lionised its role in the liberation of Zimbabwe, prioritised the centrality of the fight for land, and demonised all those outside the selective history it espoused (Raftopoulos 2009). Additionally, the party represented its stance as part of a longer lineage of pan-Africanist and anti-imperialist struggles on the African continent and globally (Ndlovu-Gatsheni 2009a). Further still, this broad line of argument indicts the ruling party for its (expensive) involvement in the war in the DRC and its unbudgeted financial support and pensions for war veterans in the late 1990s. Both of these actions have been interpreted as cynical strategies of co-optation in which the ruling party sought to consolidate its power by securing patronage networks within the military and the war veterans' association (Muzondidya 2009; Alao 2012). And crucially, ZANU (PF)'s destruction of the commercial farming sector, particularly between 2000 and 2003, marked a central watershed in the precipitation of the crisis (Hammar, Raftopoulos and Jensen 2003; Phimister and Raftopoulos 2004). Fundamentally, this body of scholarship posits that violence, rights violations, lawlessness and intolerance of political dissent were carried out to entrench the political and financial interests of the ruling party and its patrimonial beneficiaries when faced with a powerful opposition.

In the second frame, Sam Moyo and Paris Yeros adopt a 'revolutionary', self-avowed Marxist interpretation of the crisis. In fact, these scholars challenge the very notion of '[a] Zimbabwe crisis' and argue that this period of political change was in reality 'an interrupted revolution marked by a radical agrarian reform and a radicalized state', which had rebelled against neo-colonialism (Moyo and Yeros 2007a: 103). For Moyo and Yeros (2007a; 2007b), this rebellion began after 1997 when the state, under ZANU(PF), pursued a political-economic turnaround in Zimbabwe that entailed the suspension of economic structural adjustment programmes, the beginning of active state intervention in the land question, intervention in the DRC against US-backed rebels, and debt default. At that point, they argue,

Western governments and the International Financial Institutions imposed 'all the economic and political conditionalities' beginning with the suspension of balance of payments support by the World Bank, and followed by 'a broad range of formal and informal sanctions, including a sustained propaganda campaign against Zimbabwe to the point of comparing "Mugabe" to "Miloševic"' (Moyo and Yeros 2007b: 184). Critically, this perspective emphasises the tensions and contradictions of this 'revolution'. It points out that ZANU(PF)'s policies towards land and economic reforms heralded a struggle against 'imperialism' and 'neo-liberalism', but the party failed to broaden its social base and gain popular support – especially from the urban areas – when the peasants' 'revolution' was co-opted by the party's 'bourgeois interests'.

There are important limits to the extent to which this latter line of argument can be sustained. Its overemphasis on the self-interest and venality of the West downplays the authoritarianism of the ruling party, its human rights violations and its disruptive domestic actions during the crisis (Tendi 2010). Throughout much of this book, I argue in favour of the position articulated by Jocelyn Alexander (2013), who contends that one of the most significant responses of ZANU(PF) to the crisis was its 'assault' on key aspects of what had previously made Zimbabwean state bureaucracies authoritative: that is, their 'expert, rule-bound character' (Alexander 2013: 807). This assault – manifest as manipulating the law, deploying political violence and making partisan use of state institutions and resources – was, she argues, necessary to ZANU(PF)'s strategy for retaining political power.

Alexander's argument is powerfully illustrated by the politics of land reform in the late 1990s and early 2000s. During this time ZANU(PF) set out to convince the electorate that only the ruling party could rectify the historical injustice of land alienation by casting the MDC, white farmers and the British in an unholy imperial alliance intent on depriving Zimbabweans of their land. In contrast to previous state-led land resettlement programmes of the 1980s and early 1990s, in 2000 the party supported war veterans and partisan youth militia who occupied white-owned farms, often deploying violence against farmers and their workers, as a means of forcing land redistribution. In less than five years, the number of white farmers actually farming the land dwindled from about 4,500 to under 500, while as many as 200,000 farm workers had lost their jobs, and often with them their homes and access to services. ZANU(PF) equated any criticism of the occupations with belittling the country's liberation history and struggle for sovereignty, as well as the real need for land in Zimbabwe's communal areas. The combination of ZANU(PF)'s violent electioneering and the land occupations ushered in a new logic of political power that saw the transformation of the state and political sphere (Alexander 2006).

This new logic of political power both weakened and politicised the state: 'professionalism, education, and skills were no longer the predominant criteria for holding state posts; loyalty to ZANU(PF) and political and military connections were' (Alexander 2010: 195). Moreover, these changes undermined what had once been one of ZANU (PF)'s most compelling claims to legitimacy: the delivery of public services by professional civil servants. Several authors explore the changes highlighted by Alexander in specific public arenas beyond the farm including the courts (Verheul 2013), the military (Tendi 2013), the prisons (Alexander 2013) and local government (McGregor 2013). All authors underscore 'the uncomfortable articulation of contrasting, historically shaped commitments to normative constructions of statehood and political legitimacy and the heated contestation over practices of patronage, corruption and coercion that both linked and distinguished them' (Alexander and McGregor 2013: 752).

Within these rich explorations into various facets of the state in Zimbabwe and within the wider and voluminous scholarship on the country's crisis, almost no attention has been paid to public health from a social and political perspective despite three salient social and political features of the Zimbabwean health system: (1) according to UNICEF, Zimbabwe's health sector was, until the 2000s, 'one of the best in sub-Saharan Africa' (Beukes 2013); (2) healthcare delivery has historically played a critical role in buttressing the legitimacy of the ruling party (Muzondidya 2009); and (3) a public health emergency, born partly out of the 'disintegration' of the health system, was a central feature of the nadir of the crisis (J. L. Jones 2010b). At the same time, the literature on the cholera outbreak from the health sciences has not interrogated the politics of the epidemic beyond identifying 'increasing poverty, bad governance, poor economic policies, widespread HIV/AIDS, and a weakened health system' as structural drivers of the country's health crisis (Todd et al. 2009: 3). What is missing in the literature, and is provided in this book, is a socio-political account of the cholera outbreak that links the epidemic to changes in the health system and to the wider transformation of state institutions and politics.

Epidemics as Social and Political Disasters

Shifting our attention away from the state and formal structures of political order, studying the cholera outbreak takes us into various social realms that reveal how people experienced Zimbabwe's crisis at its lowest point. Throughout this book, I describe how my interlocutors make meaning out of illness and explain the cholera outbreak in terms of the social, economic and political ills afflicting the country as a whole. My theoretical approach to epidemics as social and political disasters thus links the subjective experience of illness to the political forces that socially pattern disease and that thereby reinforce or exacerbate hierarchical distinctions between different members of the body politic. I tie together three different and salient literatures to develop this line of thinking; they are: the sociology of disasters, critical medical anthropology and the anthropology of citizenship.

The first set of literatures – the sociology of disasters – is derivative of and broadly sympathetic to critical political ecology (Forsyth 2004). It accords primary significance to the social and the political elements of a disaster over the physical and the biological. Drawing on this literature, I emphasise the following. Regarding the relationship between state and society, Jennifer Rubenstein (2015) argues that disasters often accentuate the social struggles in a society and underscore the inherent inequities within a political system. Similarly, Alex de Waal (1997), in his innovative work *Famine Crimes: Politics and the Disaster Relief Industry in Africa*, explains that the way in which governmental and humanitarian sectors act in response and recovery to a disaster is largely predicated on the kind of political relationships that existed between state and society before the crisis. Furthermore, Mark Pelling and Kathleen Dill (2010) suggest that disasters are 'tipping points' or, as Vasudha Chhotray (2014: 217) puts it, 'Disasters are key political moments in the life of a society.' This view holds that disasters potentially bear new possibilities for actors to transcend the past, elide pre-existing social inequalities and reinvent the social contract. But, as Rajesh Venugopal and Sameer Yasir (2017) caution, this optimistic scenario of transformation through a political unlocking is far from typical. More frequently, disasters arouse public anger and outrage at the inadequacy of government relief efforts, and they coalesce political mobilisations about the incompetence, or the politicised distribution, of relief (Venugopal and Yasir 2017). On this latter point, the response to disasters is as important as their causes. At the heart of the larger political dynamics that follow disasters are the ways in which the provision of relief as well as the identification of blame and failure are established and translated through moral-cognitive frameworks. Thus, it is argued, those who have the capacity and willingness to visibly provide relief can potentially gain in legitimacy, gratitude, and public standing while, at the same time, those who are seen to be inactive, absent or profiting from the misery of others can potentially be legitimised. Therefore, political stakes in any disaster are high, and so alongside the competition to command and allocate resources is another, more frantic competition to shape public perceptions (Venugopal and Yasir 2017).

In sum, this literature suggests that conditions of emergency and abject human need are potential moments of reinvention or reproduction, in which political success and failure can be forged. An important criticism of this work, however, is that in its foregrounding of the political over the physical and biological it ignores the bodily experience of suffering and the concrete achievements of life-saving relief (see Scott-Smith 2014). In the case of an epidemic, as I argue repeatedly, the materiality of suffering is an integral part of both the lived experience of disaster and its wider politics.

Critical medical anthropology (CMA) helps us along further in thinking through what it means to look at epidemics as a specific kind of disaster. The subdiscipline of CMA is held together by a common, theoretical perspective that focuses on explicating or grounding health inequities in reference to constellations of political economy, regional history, noxious social conditions and development ideology (Janes and Corbett 2009). The merging of medical anthropology's focus on culture and healing systems with a more critical political economy perspective is summed up well by Allan Young (1982). In a seminal review essay, Young argues that medical anthropology's role is not merely to contextualise understandings of illness but also to demonstrate how social relations produce the forms and distribution of sickness in a given society. Similar arguments have since been advanced by several other scholars (for example, Vaughan 1991;

Scheper-Hughes 1992; Fassin 2007a; Kleinman 2010), perhaps most famously by Paul Farmer (2001a: 262) who describes infectious diseases as the 'biological expression of social inequalities'.

Sherine Hamdy (2008) takes these discussions in CMA further by arguing for the need to offer both a culturalist and a materialist view of illness and social inequality but not via the conventional anthropological division of labour. That is, Hamdy argues against a neat distinction between, on the one hand, her informants' knowledge as a 'local' or 'cultural' (subjective) understanding of illness and, on the other, her own analysis as a 'real' or 'factual' (objective) interpretation of the ways in which inequalities of power produce and distribute illness. Instead, Hamdy argues for the concept of 'political aetiologies' – the notion that pathological bodily processes are situated adjacent to pathological socio-political processes in popular accounts of witnessing and living with a calamitous disease. In her study of patients with end-stage kidney disease in Egypt, she writes: 'The connection that patients make between their illness and failed state policies is not merely abstract or cerebral; it is a connection that they experience in material and bodily forms as well' (Hamdy 2008: 561). Like Hamdy, I aimed to forge a 'collaborative alliance' with my informants, whose physical and political grievances allowed me to understand how cholera was disproportionately experienced by the poor because of particular social structures that foster environmental contamination, unsafe food and water, urban poverty and inadequate medical treatment. I appropriate Hamdy's notion of 'political aetiologies' and repurpose it to theorise the changing configurations of citizenship and political subjectivities that are born out of individual and collective suffering during and after a medical disaster. To elaborate, I now turn to the anthropological literature on citizenship and political subjectivity.

The anthropological scholarship on citizenship has grown immensely in the last two decades. This work has suggested that citizenship cannot be read simply as a formal category of belonging that assures its bearer of equal membership in a national polity (Anand 2017). Rather, it is argued that citizenship is a contingent, often flexible form of political subjectification that emerges through both iterative and constitutive interactions and performances between the state and its subjects (Ong 1996). Citizenship is therefore claimed through the formal practices of voting, as well as everyday performances of social belonging, and through demands for the resources of states. While formal citizenship promises equality among citizens, the anthropology of citizenship literature draws attention to the unequal distribution of substantive civil, political, socioeconomic, and cultural rights among individuals and how these are differentially recognised by state and/or state-like institutions (see also Holston 2008). The graduated forms of membership to the body politic that ensue demonstrate how citizenship can be inclusive, yet also dramatically unequal (Holston 2008)

Two strands of the anthropology of citizenship literature are especially relevant to the present work. The first is Nikhil Anand's concept of hydraulic citizenship. For Anand (2017: 8) hydraulic citizenship is 'the ability of residents to be recognized by city agencies through legitimate water services'. Anand argues that hydraulic citizenship is not a linear process realized through the accreted recognitions of city laws, documents and policies, or the outcome of political protest or social recognition, but rather is a cyclical, iterative process that is highly dependent on social histories, political technologies and the infrastructures of water distribution in the city (Anand 2017: 8).

Throughout the book, I show how access to public services – especially water and sanitation – is a crucial mediator of citizenship in the cyclical, iterative way highlighted by Anand. I take this analysis further by examining hydraulic citizenship in Zimbabwe during the cholera crisis and by showing what political subjectivities emerge in the process. To do this, I draw on a second salient strand of the literature on citizenship, which comes from a growing body of work that examines what kinds of citizens are produced by humanitarian emergencies, such as deadly outbreaks.

This latter literature tends to understand citizenship through the idiom of 'resilience' (Scott-Smith 2018). Emergencies, according to this literature, are no longer imagined as interruptions to progress, but presented as an opportunity to manage precariousness and risk. The task of humanitarians, and sometimes the state, when they pursue this vision of resilience, is to help individuals become robust, adaptable, entrepreneurial citizens, taking care of their own inevitably insecure futures. As Mark Duffield (2011: 23) puts it, resilience 'functions more as ideology … promoting a post-political life of constant adaptation, [and] the abandonment of long-term expectations'. And Marc Welsh (2014: 20) offers the following summary of humanitarian resilience:

> [R]esilience approaches operate on the normative assumption that communities can and should self-organise to deal with uncertainty, that uncertainty is a given not something with a political dimension, and the role of government is limited to enabling, shaping and supporting, but specifically not to direct or to fund those processes. This locates the responsibility of 'communities' as needing to organise themselves, primarily in the context of sustaining economic growth. As a consequence, there is little sign of a profound engagement with a politics of resilience as a means for conceiving of change; of revolution through resilience.

In this book, I suggest that subjective experiences of citizenship will expand our understandings of the dynamics of inclusion and exclusion from the body politic and the shifting relationships between the state and its citizens at a time of crisis. To do this, I use the term 'political subjectivity' to denote how people relate to governance and authorities; to consider how they are brought into a position to stake claims, to have a voice, and to be recognisable by authorities; and to explore how the politics of identity and belonging, encompassing the substantive as well as the judicial-political dimension of claims to citizenship, are expressed in specific contexts (Krause and Schramm 2011). With reference to the cholera epidemic, this frame of analysis considers how people stake claims to medical treatment and social welfare; how they relate to state institutions that are failing to deliver basic services effectively; and how they see themselves in relation to the body politic and what impact such imaginaries have on notions of the public good and the responsibility of the state.

Outbreaks like cholera always produce and reflect social and political difference. They mark the boundaries between social inclusion on one hand against abandonment and exclusion on the other. Citizenship is thereby actualised by situated and quotidian encounters with different institutions and officials of the state and political subjectivities are born out of these encounters. An outbreak brings such encounters with the state to vivid light in every phase and aspect of its unfolding from origins to resolution. As such, cholera, like other outbreaks, reveal how substantive citizenship is constituted: indexed by access to public services and emergency relief, and violated by anachronistic structures, such as the outdated waterworks in their community, or by the arbitrary demolition exercises of the state.

One Disease, Many Crises

In a narrow biological sense, cholera is an acute bacterial infection of the intestine caused by the ingestion of food or water contaminated by certain strains of the organism, *Vibrio cholerae* (Lee 2001). In theory, cholera should not be a major threat to humans. Not only is susceptibility highly variable between individuals, but the bacteria can only be acquired in one way: through the ingestion of food and water that has been contaminated either by faecal matter from a person with active cholera, or from free-standing bacteria present in plankton or seafood living in infected brackish water (Echenberg 2011). An authoritative article, published in 1976 in *The Johns Hopkins Medical Journal*, has been widely cited in cholera research for noting that, in terms of pathophysiology, cholera causes 'only a reversible and easily treatable biochemical defect,' and for claiming that cholera requires 'a very gross level of contamination, greater than for any other known epidemic disease' to produce illness in normal individuals (Carpenter 1976). Clinically, this accounts for why cholera rarely infects healthcare workers involved in its treatment. While many individuals will only acquire asymptomatic or mild cases of cholera, the disease's progress is frightening for those who are more susceptible. In the following paragraphs, I summarise the clinical course of cholera (see Echenberg 2011).

Incubation – the period between exposure to the pathogen and the manifestation of symptoms and signs – ranges from as short as fourteen hours to as long as five days. The variation depends on how long it takes for the cholera *vibrios* to colonise and multiply in the small intestine after they enter the body. In the intestine, the bacteria secrete a powerful toxin that interferes with colonic absorption of water, salts and other electrolytes. As a result, the first stage of symptoms includes sudden and explosive watery diarrhoea – classically called 'rice water stool' – that gushes out of the patient, emptying the lower bowel of faecal matter quickly. In a single day, an individual patient can pass up to twenty litres of stool containing as many as ten million *vibrios* per millilitre. This frequent and painless diarrhoea is accompanied by hiccups, extensive retching and vomitus of the same whitish appearance, which may contain cholera bacteria. The tremendous loss of water and electrolytes can amount to 8 per cent loss of normal body weight. The consequent dehydration produces acute and agonising cramps in the muscles of the feet and legs, and occasionally the arms, abdomen and back. The sense of prostration is often extreme, lasting from 2 to 12 hours, depending on the severity of the symptoms.

The second stage, often reached in a day or two, is marked by continued purging and vomiting, and then collapse. Rapid dehydration and ruptured capillaries lend an ashen appearance to the patient. The skin becomes blue and black, cold, wrinkled and clammy to the touch; the voice becomes husky; the cheeks hollow; the eyes sunken; and the expression listless. Signs of hypovolaemic shock (a severe state of decreased blood volume) appear: the blood pressure falls, a pulse is not palpable at the wrist, and urine output is suppressed. The legs and stomach convulse violently causing terrible pain. Loss of body fluids is often so great that blood can run as thickly as tar, while puncturing a vein – for a blood test or to insert an intravenous line – produces no results. All the while, the patient suffers the horror of cholera often with full consciousness of her or his plight. Without adequate fluid replacement, death can occur from circulatory shock, due to low blood perfusion of vital tissues and organs, or kidney failure. In the most dramatic cases, a healthy person can die within hours.

A third stage, for those who survive this critical attack, ultimately brings a cessation of vomiting and diarrhoea. If the second stage can be limited to only a few hours, then it is possible to restore circulation and blood pressure and the flow of urine will resume. It may seem that recovery is assured at this point. However, death can still occur within four or five days should impaired kidney function develop.

In terms of cholera treatment, clinical trials for an effective vaccine have been under way since the 1990s, but by far the most important development in this respect has been the ability to rehydrate patients quickly and effectively by means of an inexpensive intervention, oral rehydration therapy (ORT). Indeed, ORT has, over the past three decades, become one of the greatest success stories in the chronicles of modern medicine. ORT entails the administration of gentle concoctions containing sugar, salts and other products and it is as simple and inexpensive to deliver as it is effective. When delivered correctly, ORT can reduce mortality from cholera to less than 1 per cent. Given that ORT, a simple therapeutic tool, is readily and cheaply available worldwide, cholera is not only preventable; it is eminently treatable. No one should die of cholera today (Echenberg 2011).

Considering this, the emergence of cholera is always troubling. Throughout the intellectual history of epidemiology, Charles Rosenberg (1992: 293) identifies two fundamental styles of explanation of an epidemic's seemingly random incursions into society that have been conceptually 'available' since classical antiquity. He labels these alternative styles *contamination* and *configuration*. Contamination typically reduces itself to the idea of person-to-person contagion, that is, the transmission of some morbid material from one individual to another. The configuration theme, by contrast, is 'holistic and emphasises system, interconnection, and balance, while the contamination foregrounds a particular disordering element' (Rosenberg 1992: 203). Where the configurational style of explanation is interactive, contextual and often environmental, the emphasis on contamination is reductionist and monocausal. I argue that cholera epidemics can only be understood through a configurational style of explanation. Since the disease is primarily transmitted through food and water, is difficult to spread and is easily prevented, it only tends to appear in epidemic form in contexts where people are living in overcrowded and dilapidated housing or temporary settlements; where sanitary conditions are poor; and where malnutrition is widespread and severe. As such, cholera outbreaks are rare in the absence of major structural change such as war or catastrophic environmental events. In other words, cholera outbreaks often result from and then compound a social, economic and/or political disaster.

At an individual level, cholera is terrifying given the truly horrible suffering that the disease can inflict on its victims. Deeply lodged in the collective memory of many cultures globally, cholera's association with violent purging of both faeces and vomit evokes revulsion and shame in both patients and caregivers (Arnold 1986; Briggs and Mantini-Briggs 2004; Evans 2006). The inability to control the bladder and bowels in the process of bodily elimination of waste is inscribed in different ways throughout the life course: as a natural sign of infancy in the early years of life; as a humiliating sign of dependency in adulthood; and as a morbid sign of senility in old age (Echenberg 2011). At a social level, cholera is 'the quintessential disease of filth' (Echenberg 2011: 9), and this association, much more so than its potential and real lethality, helps to explain why it triggers such powerful popular reactions. From as far back as the late eighteenth century, the symptoms of cholera involved bodily functions that were hidden from public view in 'respectable' Western society, and those who engaged in such practices – degraded as marginals, vagrants, drunkards or the mentally ill – were disqualified from 'civilised' society. Politically, cholera is a manifestation of infrastructural breakdown and the failure to provide adequate sanitation, hygiene and medical care.

The label epidemic – 'the occurrence in a community of an illness, specific health-related behavior, or other health-related events clearly in excess of normal expectancy' (Last 2001: 60) – has divergent meanings for different individuals and communities experiencing the phenomenon, and it is always situated in a particular set of material conditions shaped by local, national and global processes. The technical definition of an epidemic fails to capture this complexity and instead tends to homogenise, erase and belie the diversity of experiences of people who are suffering or have suffered through what we call epidemics (Herring and Swedlund 2010). In large part, this stems from the seemingly neutral statistical language of counting, so fundamental to the science of epidemiology and to the definition of 'epidemic', which aims to establish an authoritative analysis, a process of knowledge accumulation and the systematic application of that knowledge to public health problems. Such a technocratic worldview dismisses the political as 'subjective', and instead finds safe haven in the certainties, measurability and rationality of the 'objective' (Jasanoff 2004).

There is a long tradition in social science of critiquing positivist approaches to knowing epidemics by pluralising the epistemologies of disease and investigating how epidemics have been interpreted, understood and remembered in the intellectual context of their time (see, for example, Rosenberg 1989, 1992; Vaughan 1991; Ranger and Slack 1995; Comaroff 2007; Herring and Swedlund 2010). While such contributions form part of the intellectual foundations of this book, it remains the case that what has been explored to a lesser degree in social science are the theoretical implications of how epidemics are 'handled in practice' (Mol 2002: 5). If we take an epidemic as our analytical object and travel with it as it is handled in practice from one site to the next, a new series of insights about epidemics emerges. We find that one disease is linked to many crises.

From the laboratory to the clinic, from the household to the community, from the refugee camp to the boardroom, the reality of cholera takes a variety of forms. The medical anthropologist and philosopher

Annemarie Mol (1999; 2002) would describe this multiplicity as cholera's 'multiple ontologies'. It is more than a straightforward biological infection. Cholera is a microorganism, a disease, an epidemic, an illness, a public health crisis, a social disaster and a political scandal at the same time. Moreover, there are no rigid boundaries between these different forms of cholera; they are frequently interdependent. They exist in the same universe, sometimes in harmony, sometimes in conflict. Apprehending the politics of cholera is, in a fundamental way, an exercise in ontological politics – the politics of what is real and how these different realities co-exist and collide with each other. The realities of cholera are historically, culturally and materially located.

Cholera is a corporeal phenomenon. People see its clinical signs. They smell the waste it produces. They touch bodies stricken by the disease. It causes physical pain and emotional distress. Experiencing cholera shapes how people act on it whether in the laboratory, on the ward or at a meeting. In an interview, Tendai Biti, the Minister of Finance in Zimbabwe's Government of National Unity between 2009 and 2013, described the cholera crisis as 'visceral': 'This crisis was physical, unlike now. It's one of the differences between 2008 and now. Right now, the crisis is not physical. You don't see it.'[1]

In my theoretical schema, reality is not only imagined, it is also 'done'; it is not only observed, it is also enacted. Instead of attributes or aspects, there are different, yet related, versions of the cholera outbreak. The reality of the epidemic cannot be held in clear-cut contradistinction from perspectives and narratives. Rather it is immanent in social practices, identities, norms, conventions, instruments and institutions (Jasanoff 2004). Furthermore, there is also a politics to this multiplicity. After all, the multiplicity of cholera is not endless; it exists in and is bounded by time, place, context and history. It has specific effects. It entails conflict and choices.

The 'one disease, many crises' framework helps to explain why epidemics are such sites of struggle. It highlights the limitations of an exclusively positivist understanding of epidemics; it takes bodily experiences of disease seriously as much as it pays attention to the ways in which knowledge about epidemics is socially constructed and challenged. I map out the following general features of an epidemic's multiple ontologies, which serve as a theoretical guide through this

[1] Interview, Tendai Biti, Harare, 16 November 2015.

book. Epidemics are biological phenomena, an infectious disease spreading through a given population in excess of normal expectancy. Epidemics are social phenomena. They spread through populations in socially patterned ways as noxious socio-material conditions interact with the biological properties of an infectious disease to make epidemics virulent among specific vulnerable groups in a population. Epidemics are historical phenomena. They are not random incursions into everyday life, but rather are the culmination of multi-scalar, political-economic processes that obtain over time. Epidemics are political phenomena. The declaration of an epidemic is a social, not a scientific, claim. It is made by actors and institutions against a set of background conditions to given audiences, who then accept, ignore, challenge or reject that claim. Moreover, the declaration of an epidemic is almost always followed by political contests over the attention, resources and priority that said epidemic should receive.

Tying all these threads together then, this book is about the causes and consequences of the cholera outbreak. It is about the many different forms that cholera took. It is about the multiple ways that people encountered and responded to cholera. It is about how cholera shaped people's understandings of politics and their individual and collective positions in Zimbabwean society. And it is about how people remember the outbreak and speak of their experiences.

Methodology

I examined the origins of the cholera outbreak, the manner of its unfolding, the lived experience of the disease and its attendant political subjectivities through a range of different sources. Of central importance were the stories that people told about the outbreak. I suggest that the retelling of experiences of the outbreak is significant not only for bringing hitherto undocumented narratives to light but also for what such retelling says of those narrators themselves and of the way that the cholera disaster has been committed to historical memory (Ranger and Slack 1995; Briggs and Mantini-Briggs 2004; Venugopal and Yasir 2017). I make the case that the telling of stories is always a political act and, in this way, stories are an especially illuminating prism through which to explore the politics and social contours of the cholera outbreak and its aftermath. Nikhil Anand (2017) writes that stories have multiple vocalities and multiple sites of production.

Unlike discourses, he contends, stories are finely attuned to the diverse locations at which human agency is hampered, but they also present other ways of knowing the world. In this sense, storytelling is a vital human strategy for sustaining agency in the face of circumstances that the storytellers view as disempowering (see also Jackson 2002). Furthermore, the act of reconstituting events in a story means that one is no longer living those events in passivity but is actively reworking them in dialogue with others and within one's own imagination. The dialogical character of storytelling reveals the intricate relation between individual and collective memory as a complex composite, neither entirely ineffable and individual nor entirely socially determined (Nuttall 1998).

My work has much in common with Charles Briggs's (2004) exploration of the manifold meanings of cholera in the wake of the 1992–93 epidemic on the Orinoco Delta of Venezuela. In *Stories in the Time of Cholera: Racial Profiling during a Medical Nightmare*, Briggs argues that illness narratives told during and after epidemics may help people to cope with the search for order that takes place when sickness shatters their perspectives on daily life (c.f. Jackson 2002). However, competing narratives characterise the same events in quite different ways thereby inviting highly contrasting sorts of remedial action. In Briggs's case study, cholera created a charged, high-stakes debate about the lives of the people it infected, and competing stories bore quite different policy and, of course, political implications. As he (Briggs 2004: 7) puts it,

> Each cholera story created a dramatis personae, a series of events, and a set of causal inferences, casting some parties as heroes who acted wisely and courageously, others as villains who promoted death for gain or glory, and still others as pathetic bystanders not smart enough to get out of the way … It is, of course, not simply the content of cholera narratives that rendered them potent. … In examining the mechanisms through which stories were produced, transmitted, imbued with legitimacy, and challenged, we see that narratives had very real effects on how people lived and died.

As in Briggs's work so it is in this study that the cholera stories people told varied widely. Despite their many differences, narrators tended to view the epidemic in terms of its broad social, political and historical factors – that is, in terms of its political aetiologies. The epidemic variably took its place among stories of failed governance, political conflict, human rights violations, environmental degradation and institutional corruption. How people had hitherto experienced Zimbabwe's political-economic crisis deeply affected how they perceived and reacted to the disease. Cholera was cast in some of these narratives as the unintentional but inevitable by-product of broad political, economic and social forces; in others it was a weapon of mass destruction used intentionally to finish the job – after organised political violence – of punishing the urban poor for their allegiance to opposition politicians.

The cholera epidemic and the stories told about it point to the crucial importance of people's relationships to medicine, public health, humanitarian organisations, political parties, physical infrastructure and the state. The stories of cholera are co-constitutive of its politics. They are about claims to legitimacy and social standing, they are about anger and recrimination, they are about ideologies and historical consciousness.

Writing about the social experience of disasters is a vexing task. Such narratives exhibit multiple logics, styles and mutations that relate to each other through mediation, contradiction and transformation (Choi 2013). Any attempt to render such multifarious stories legible is unavoidably an act of realist fiction. What I offer in this work is not an objective account about the cholera outbreak but a subjective one based on my own intellectual choices (and limitations) and by the practical conditions in which I gathered my data. Accepting these limitations at the outset, I explain how I grappled methodologically with such a dense and intricate subject matter.

I pursued my research qualitatively through multiple avenues of inquiry including formal interviews, informal conversations, focus group discussions, visits to relevant institutions and field sites, and examination of primary and secondary materials. Discussing cholera frequently stoked painful memories for many of my interlocutors. It was thus imperative for me to build trust and establish my credibility as a committed scholar through numerous conversations, often informal, with key informants before progressing to detailed and in-depth discussions about what happened during the 2008–09 outbreak. In many instances, focus group discussions were the chosen format, as a large number of my informants in Harare's high-density townships felt more at ease discussing the horrors of 2008–09 in a group rather than individually. The range of conversational and interview styles through which I learnt about the outbreak and uncovered memories about it allowed me to triangulate information iteratively before arriving at theoretical saturation. Speaking to a variety of people formally and informally, individually and collectively proved highly effective as a means of tracing the different historical processes that led to the cholera outbreak, of understanding how different actors experienced and responded to the disease, and for elucidating the political debates, popular narratives and power struggles it provoked.

I interpreted my data iteratively and according to the principles of 'grounded theory' – using systematic, inductive procedures to generate insights grounded in the views expressed by the study participants (Glaser and Strauss 1967). Practically, during the primary period of fieldwork between July 2015 and January 2016, this meant that I adopted an evolving project design wherein I identified key informants firstly through known channels (such as contacting relevant institutions) and then subsequently through 'snowballing' as many of my interviewees directed me to other individuals who were well placed to speak to my research questions. 'Snowballing' opened multiple avenues of research for me; however, in the high-density townships this method did limit me to certain social networks – often with similar political inclinations and experiences – thereby limiting the inferences I can make about the township population more generally.

I conducted 75 individual and group interviews with 125 people. My interviewees can loosely be grouped together around my different research questions. In the high-density townships and communities that were epicentres of the outbreak, I conducted a series of in-depth individual and group interviews. I examined how these urbanites experienced and interpreted the outbreak and how this influenced, if at all, their relationships to institutions of governance and authority, particularly at a time of deepening impoverishment and in the aftermath of the worst political violence in the post-2000 period in Zimbabwe (Alexander and Chitofiri 2010). I also conducted interviews with people involved in various facets of the response to the outbreak such as the medical and humanitarian, the long-term developmental, and the human rights and legal. In these discussions, I explored different perspectives on the origins of the outbreak as well as the forms of responsibility, civic commitments and collectives that animated the configurations of health care delivery and intervention and that organised claims to health-related human rights. Relatedly, I looked at how different actors, embedded in these varied organisational entities, interpreted the actions of the central government, under the aegis of the ruling party. In addition, I met with current and former politicians and civil servants in the Ministries of Health, Local Government and Finance. I interviewed politicians in opposition parties who were politically involved in trying to address the cholera outbreak. I asked my interlocutors how they understood the cholera outbreak within the wider context of Zimbabwe's political crisis and what impact the epidemic had on their priorities, policies, and decision-making. I also examined the discursive and material strategies deployed by the ruling party to assert its political dominance at a time when its legitimacy was being contested and, more generally, I explored how officials spoke of their individual and institutional roles during the cholera crisis. Overall, my informants in this study represent a wide range of different backgrounds in terms of age, education, ethnicity, location, occupation and political orientation.

Throughout the book, I rely heavily on direct quotes from my interviews to emphasise and privilege the voices and perspectives of my interlocutors. In many cases, I have anonymised the identity of my informants through use of an alias, either because they did not wish to be named or because I felt that they shared politically sensitive information that potentially compromised their safety. I use ambiguity as a protective measure for the identity of my informants by not making clear when I have used a real name or an alias. Unless otherwise stated, the quotes chosen encapsulate sentiments expressed by multiple other respondents. It is for the sake of brevity, clarity and coherence that, where several informants express the same idea, I foreground an illustrative utterance.

Finally, and in addition to my interviews, I collated an extensive catalogue of documentary sources. I sourced journalistic accounts of the 2008–09 cholera outbreak from the online archives of major global media organisations and from the physical archives of *The Herald*, Zimbabwe's national newspaper, in Harare. While I was unable to access the physical archives of independent newspapers in Zimbabwe, I managed to interview several independent journalists and senior editors. Other key sources included publicly available minutes of meetings, policy papers, technical reports and post-outbreak evaluations from UN agencies (notably UNICEF, WHO, United Nations Office for the Coordination of Humanitarian Affairs) and the IOM as well as from policy think tanks, NGOs and other civil society and advocacy groups. Human rights and humanitarian investigations conducted during the outbreak, particularly by Physicians for Human Rights and the International Crisis Group, offer detailed accounts of conditions on the ground and therefore receive close attention and analysis in the book.

Like any book, this work has important limitations. Conducted in retrospect, I was deprived of the ethnographic perspective. As Darryl Stellmach (2016) has noted, catastrophes can be invisible, they can unfold imperceptibly. In order to identify a disaster as it happens, responders of various kinds balance imperfect and competing data, motivations and imperatives, and often identification and response happen simultaneously. By corollary, responses to catastrophes are never fully coherent, with action changing constantly in reaction to new data and new developments. Studying a catastrophe that has already happened means that events that were, at one time, very difficult to interpret have now fully declared their salience. Thus, the stories I have gathered and represent in the book clearly reflect recrimination, outrage and blame over such issues as delayed action when at the time the situation may have looked different. This is almost impossible to know for sure in retrospect.

An important aspect of the cholera outbreak that does not appear in this book regards medical pluralism. A combination of fear of stigma and the desire to appear 'respectable' and 'modern' most likely means that many of my informants did not volunteer their experiences of seeking out traditional healers during the outbreak. It should not be surprising if my own status as a foreign-educated, Westernised medical doctor did not invite such openness.

Nevertheless, the data gathered elucidate the political economy of the cholera outbreak, the myriad crises that the epidemic gave rise to, the dynamics of change in Zimbabwe's state institutions and the politics of humanitarian agencies in response to the disease.

The Argument in Brief

In this book, I make three interlocking arguments. First, I make an argument about Zimbabwe's bureaucratic state and the changes in the country's political order. I posit that the cholera epidemic was not an isolated, 'shocking' moment but, in an analogous way to famine (see de

Waal 1989; Keen 1991), it was the final stage of drawn-out, contingent processes rooted in questions of political economy such as the inadequate delivery of public goods, failing livelihood strategies and profound social inequalities. In this sense, it was a 'man-made' disaster albeit one whose making was protracted and path-dependent, determined by real historical decisions and non-decisions, and in political conflicts. The cholera outbreak brings new perspective to bear on the trajectory of the state in Zimbabwe and the post-2000 crisis. It shows, in graphic and painful detail, how the ruling party's strategies for retaining political power both devastated public infrastructures and undermined bureaucratic institutions, and how these changes interacted in a synergistic and toxic way to bring about a public health catastrophe. Cholera throws into sharp relief the interconnections between different facets of Zimbabwe's crisis and, more generally, this book shows how an epidemic is produced by and reproduces multiple crises.

Second, by carefully detailing the vast and divergent range of experiences of Zimbabwe's cholera outbreak in this book, I bring to light the epidemic's multiple ontologies. These multiple ontologies engendered fraught and contentious politics as different organisational entities, communities and individuals collided with each other in their attempts to command the narrative about cholera and shape the response to it according to their respective ideologies, institutional mandates and political ambitions. Furthermore, I argue that through a combination of the multiple ontologies of cholera, the nature of the humanitarian response to it, and the wider context of political disruption, violence and crisis in Zimbabwe, the cholera outbreak – despite being such a disaster – was not a 'tipping point' in the country's social and political life. The multiple ontologies precluded a shared understanding of the outbreak and its causes. Instead, they contributed to a political impasse – one that did not allow for an enduring structural transformation of areas that remain vulnerable to diarrhoeal disease outbreaks through the full provision of housing rights, access to clean water and sanitation, and infrastructural improvements. These challenges were compounded by the humanitarian response. The patchwork of organisations stitched together to deal with the outbreak ultimately focused their attention on its short-term palliation, not on long-term development, public health provision or political accountability for the crisis.

While I fully recognise the exigency of saving lives, I lament the failure of a more ambitious project of transformation.

Third, I make an argument about historical memory and political subjectivity. I argue that the multiple ontologies of cholera appeared in my informants' narratives as they committed the epidemic to historical memory as a health crisis, a political-economic crisis and a social crisis, as well as a crisis of expectations, history and social identity. The political subjectivities that have emerged through and after the cholera outbreak are numerous, but I emphasise three recurring themes. I show how the disease and its attendant socio-material processes became an important site of evaluating the legitimacy of the state, of venting anger at ZANU(PF)'s manifest failings and of 'making do' (J. L. Jones 2010b) when the state was unable or unwilling to deliver. Residents of Harare's high-density townships spoke of the state in sinister terms: as an entity capable of punishing portions of the citizenry through a deadly disease and/or capable of neglecting them in times of dire need (a politics of disposability). At the same time, township residents as well as doctors, civil servants, NGO workers and others still articulated a strong normative belief about the state's role as primary provider of public goods (a politics of expectation). In their different ways, many of my informants adopted a range of survival strategies to negotiate their way through the cholera outbreak and the wider crisis (a politics of adaptation). Cholera thus instantiated the politics of disposability, of expectation and of adaptation as political subjectivities.

Anatomy of the Book

The remainder of the book unfolds as follows. Chapter 1, 'The Making of Urban (Dis)Order: Situating the Cholera Outbreak in Historical Perspective', delineates the long-term factors that predisposed Harare's townships to a diarrhoeal disease outbreak and the short-term factors that precipitated the 2008–09 cholera epidemic. Foundational to my argument is the claim that urban order in the city has always been bound up with strategies of political control and social inequality. Under colonial rule, historically produced segregation and social inequality laid down the underlying physical conditions in the high-density townships – namely poor sanitation facilities, inadequate clean water provision and overcrowded housing – for the potential spread of an epidemic in the high-density areas of the city. These conditions can be traced as far back as the late nineteenth century when Harare was founded as an administrative centre for the white settler regime. They have persisted through the twentieth century and were never adequately rectified by the post-colonial government despite its ostensible attempts to transform urban spaces in the 1980s and 1990s. Finally, the chapter examines how the post-2000 political and economic meltdown triggered an urban crisis that ultimately precipitated the cholera outbreak.

Chapter 2, '"When People Eat Shit": Cholera and the Collapse of the Zimbabwe's Public Health Infrastructure', builds on the preceding one by presenting a close analysis of the institutional and infrastructural factors that precipitated the outbreak and that perpetuated its spread. Precipitating describes the factors that immediately triggered the outbreak, while perpetuating describes the factors that maintained propitious conditions for the ongoing transmission of cholera and that curtailed an effective public health response. I argue that the origins, scale and impact of the cholera outbreak were overdetermined by a multi-level failure of Zimbabwe's public health infrastructure. I situate this multi-level failure in the country's political conflicts and economic crisis, which created a 'perfect storm' for the fulmination of cholera. The chapter is organised around three principal features of Zimbabwe's health infrastructure: the collapse of functioning healthcare delivery services; the spectacular mismanagement and sabotage of the country's water reticulation systems; and the livelihood changes ushered in by the Zimbabwe's economic meltdown and hyperinflation, which rendered vast swathes of the population vulnerable to cholera through food insecurity and malnutrition.

Chapter 3, 'Emergency Politics: Cholera as a National Disaster', begins the discussion about cholera's multiple ontologies as different actors claimed that the outbreak was an emergency based on different evaluations of what kind of emergency it was. Thus, I explore the manifold ways in which the epidemic became a terrain of polarised political struggles at national and international levels in the areas of humanitarianism, security and governance. This polarisation reached extreme levels. On the one hand, the main opposition party, the Movement for Democratic Change (MDC), along with prominent outside observers – including the International Crisis Group and a high-level panel convened by Physicians for Human Rights – described cholera as the result of 'the systematic violation of a wide range of human rights' and evidence of a 'failing' state under the stewardship of the ruling party, ZANU(PF). By contrast, elements of the Zimbabwean government decried the outbreak as racist 'biological warfare' from the West intended to bring about regime change. Through the allocation of culpability for the cholera outbreak, I argue that a more fundamental political debate about power and legitimacy to govern was taking place as evidenced by international accusations of 'state failure' vis-à-vis nationalist claims to 'state sovereignty'. Furthermore, I argue that this polarisation was deleterious in the extreme because it delayed the humanitarian relief effort, promoted non-engagement between the Zimbabwean and Western governments, and narrowed down the avenues for third-party diplomatic mediation.

Chapter 4, 'The Salvation Agenda: Medical Humanitarianism and the Response to Cholera', looks at the functioning, politics and experiences of the extraordinary assemblage of institutions and individuals that ultimately constituted the emergency response to cholera. The process of coordinating a large-scale humanitarian relief effort was riven with competing claims to leadership, authority and legitimacy within and between different government and humanitarian bodies. However, as I argue in this chapter, these heterogeneous positions converged on the ineluctable and morally unimpeachable logic of 'saving lives'. I call this logic *the salvation agenda*. The salvation agenda represented a bottom-line agreement that reconciled competing experiences of and viewpoints about the crisis, to offer necessary and vital palliation in the face of cholera. Nevertheless, the exigency of saving lives did not, and could not, address the background socio-economic conditions that led to the epidemic. As such, I suggest that the salvation agenda inadvertently helped to perpetuate and, in some ways, exacerbate existing social hierarchies in Zimbabwe while ceding 'moral ownership' of the outbreak to a technical, internationalised, ostensibly ethical and apolitical humanitarian apparatus.

Chapter 5, '"People Were Dying Like Flies": The Social Contours of Cholera in Harare's Urban Townships', focuses on the views of residents in the townships where the epidemic first fulminated. My interviewees in this portion of society describe the ZANU(PF) regime in sinister terms. For them, the government has both the capacity and the willingness to inflict harm on them through a ferocious disease or to ignore them in times of desperate need. In describing their lives as disposable during and in the aftermath of this deadly illness, cholera made clear just how marginalised they are in Zimbabwean society. My interlocutors recounted stories of relentless suffering, violence, dispossession and abandonment during the cholera outbreak. It is tempting to read this grim narration as a form of victimhood – the surrender of agency – when faced with a sinister political regime and a deadly disease outbreak. But to do so, I argue, would be to grasp only one aspect of what are layered public narratives. By examining the ways in which people spoke about cholera, I underscore the limitations that 'the state' has in commanding its own discursive representations and in shaping popular understandings of a political disaster. It is here, in the recounting of the cholera outbreak, that I show the agency of my interlocutors. While they speak from an apparent position of victimhood, the outbreak also provided an occasion for township residents to vent their outrage at the government and demand better-quality, more accountable public service delivery. These were claims to substantive forms of citizenship. Moreover, I argue that for all the suffering caused by cholera outbreak, for all the chaos heralded by Zimbabwe's political-economic crisis, and for all the humanitarian intervention delivered by different actors, we see a remarkable adaptation to such circumstances.

'Conclusion: More to Admire Than to Despise?' synthesises the main arguments made in the book. I discuss how the study of the cholera outbreak has been used to illuminate a wider set of questions ranging from the character of the Zimbabwean state, the nature of structural inequalities in Zimbabwean society, ideational formations in everyday life, and the myriad meanings, memories and narratives the epidemic has left in its wake across public institutions and in civic life. I put forward the contributions that this project makes to scholarly debates about the emergence of catastrophic epidemics and the transformation of state institutions in Zimbabwe, about the politics of responding to epidemics and complex emergencies, and about citizenship and political subjectivity. I place the cholera outbreak in comparative perspective by suggesting how the insights gleaned from this book might be relevant to other major epidemics in Africa, notably the 2014 Ebola outbreak in Sierra Leone, Liberia and Guinea. Finally,

I end the book on a cautionary note, as Zimbabwe remains at risk of further diarrhoeal disease outbreaks, which continue to disproportionately affect the poor. But I also note that the country's politics are not a foregone conclusion, and despite the pessimistic tone of this book, reasons for optimism are to be found in the complexity, diversity and richness of Zimbabwean people and society.

1 The Making of Urban (Dis)Order

Situating the Cholera Outbreak in Historical Perspective

Epidemics do not just happen. They are not random events. They have histories.

—Tony Barnett and Alan Whiteside, *AIDS in the Twenty-First Century: Disease and Globalization*, 2002

Cholera is only a different shade on the canvas of ill-health. The cause of cholera is not to be found in biology, but in poverty. Inadequate and non-existent sanitation and the lack of piped clean water are the immediate causes of the spread of the disease. But the roots of cholera lie in an unequal distribution of resources – too much for some, very little or next to nothing for others.

—Dr Gerry Coovadia, *Sunday Times (Johannesburg)*, 1982

In October 2016, fully eight years after the cholera catastrophe of 2008, the Zimbabwean government issued an ominous alert about a potential cholera outbreak in multiple areas throughout the country. The Minister of the Environment, Oppah Muchinguri-Kashiri, held a press conference in which she told journalists that government was debating whether to declare 'the whole country a water shortage area' (cited in News24 2016). The announcement came less than twenty-four hours after the Minister of Health, David Parirenyatwa, publicly discussed the high risks of waterborne diseases in the event of flash floods – a common experience during Zimbabwe's rainy season. Muchinguri-Kashiri went on to add:

> Something has gone wrong with us Zimbabweans. Zimbabweans are living dangerously. We cannot live luxuriously like this and forget that we are humans ... Murungu anga akaipa asi aive noruzivo nezvemagariro emativi mana ake (The white person was cruel, but had vast knowledge on how to live in a community and care for its surroundings). (cited in News24 2016)

According to the minister, Zimbabwe had become so filthy that even the Rhodesian regime, cruel and authoritarian as it was, had managed the urban environment more hygienically and knowledgeably than contemporary Zimbabweans. She bemoaned a lack of general cleanliness throughout the whole country saying that 'Zimbabwe had become one of the dirtiest countries in Southern Africa.' As part of a cycle of self-destruction, Muchinguri-Kashiri said, Zimbabweans had become 'reckless and careless about their environment', rural communities cut down trees in farmlands randomly and without due regard for why the trees might be needed, urban dwellers pollute the environment with abandon, and, for more than a decade, raw sewage flowed through city streets while people inexplicably expected to be immune from disease. The prospect of cholera was invoked as a reminder of the deadly consequences of filth and recklessness, of the failure of people to maintain their surrounding environment. Muchinguri-Kashiri's statements gesture toward history in an ambivalent way that captures, on one hand, a sense of inherited social and environmental order from colonial rule and, on the other, a rupture in historical consciousness in which a collective sense of order and responsibility has given way to self-centredness, short-termism and disregard. Hers is a narrative of irresponsible citizenship and individual blame that belies the extended, multi-scalar political-economic factors that produce cholera epidemics.

A growing body of literature uncovers and dissects the deep historical complexity of differing, overlapping and entangled African urban imaginaries, aspirations to modernity, and notions of respectability, cutting across the divisions of class, age, gender, religion and political allegiance across urban Zimbabwe (see Raftopoulos and Yoshikuni 1999; Ranger 2007; Yoshikuni 2007; Fontein 2009; Dorman 2015). Ideas about what defines order and what constitutes filth have long been shaped by the politics of governing the city and the strategies that different authorities have used over time to deliver urban services, to regulate hygiene and waste management, to manage public housing and transport, and to police social conduct and punish deviance. These ideas give Muchinguri-Kashiri's remarks some context, but they must also be explored in relation to the material factors that underpin urban order. Infrastructure plays a central role in this regard. It is significant that Harare's hydraulic infrastructure, for instance, was first established and extended during its time as a colonial city. The production of water systems in the city was designed to discriminate between white settlers accorded full membership to the polity and Africans for whom the promises of citizenship were deferred or denied (see Anand 2017). The infrastructures that were rapidly produced, extended and renovated from late 1800s through much of the early twentieth century – roads, sanitary infrastructures, marketplaces, nascent industries and housing provision – enabled a series of constitutive, though contested, divisions necessary for the operation of racial segregation in everyday life. The social differences enabled by urban infrastructures were reproduced by the accreted laws, policies and techniques for governing the city.

The making of the 2008 cholera outbreak is bound up with the history of Harare's infrastructure and the politics of creating urban order. In this chapter, I situate the cholera outbreak in this historical perspective. I emphasise the temporal depth of the processes that led to its occurrence. I do so first by delineating the structural factors that predisposed Harare's townships to a diarrhoeal disease outbreak. Central to my argument is the claim that historically produced segregation in the name of creating urban order resulted in profound social inequality and laid down the underlying physical conditions in the high-density townships – namely poor sanitation facilities, inadequate clean water provision and other public amenities, and overcrowded housing – for the potential spread of an epidemic in these parts of the city. Such conditions can be traced as far back as the late nineteenth century when Harare was founded as a colonial administrative centre. Second, I show how these conditions have persisted through the twentieth century and were never adequately rectified by the postcolonial government, itself pursuing a contradictory and contested vision of urban order. Finally, I look more closely at shifts in Harare's urban politics during the country's post-2000 political and economic meltdown, to set the scene of 'the crisis' which precipitated the cholera outbreak (see Hammar, Raftopoulos and Jensen 2003; Raftopoulos 2009; J. L. Jones 2010b; Alexander and McGregor 2013; Dorman 2016).

Unlike the chapters that follow, which all concentrate on a very narrow timeframe pivoted around the cholera outbreak itself, this chapter takes a broader view. As such, I will touch on critical events and periods in Zimbabwe's twentieth-century history, about which there is intense scholarly debate, though I do not weigh in on these arguments. This chapter insists that a long-range view offers a crucial explanatory dimension – specifically the historical politics of urban order and infrastructure – to the events, understandings, actions and structures that defined the cholera outbreak. I must stress that I am not suggesting that the cholera outbreak was in any way inevitable, quite the opposite: by providing this historical context, I am able to show in these first two chapters of the book both the path dependency and the contingency that led to the epidemic at such an epic scale in 2008 rather than at any other time in history.

Establishing Urban Order: The City and the Colonial Frontier

At his inaugural lecture when taking a chair in the Department of History at the University of Zimbabwe, Professor David Beach (1999: 14) acerbically quipped that, 'Unfortunately, when it comes to long-term planning *Homo sapiens zimbabweansis* is not significantly different from *H. sapiens rhodesiensis*. Indeed, the two are far more alike than many would care to concede.' Beach proceeded to note that nowhere was this clearer than in the siting of what was then Salisbury, the capital city of Southern Rhodesia, by the colonial state. As he put it (Beach 1999: 14),

> Even urban planning was atrociously bad. Leaving aside the lack of thinking that left only a 45° segment of Salisbury for the African population; the very siting of the city was and is incompetent. It is well known that in 1890 the site was chosen at very short notice but what is not generally known is that in 1891 the Company (British South Africa Company) did think of re-siting it, considering Norton, Mvurwi, Darwendale and even Rusape. The proposal to move the town was rejected, allegedly because the other sites were a few metres lower and thus less healthy, but actually because six brick buildings had already been put up, and the property developers did not want to lose their investments. Consequently, the town remained where the city is, upstream of its main water supply, and thus we are condemned to drink our own recycled waste!

Beach (1999: 14) pointed out that on the eve of the new millennium, the population in Zimbabwean cities, such as Harare, was potentially increasing 'at a rate faster than the national average [and that] they are going to run short of water relatively quickly'. Muchaparara Musemwa (2012: 4) traces the post-2000 urban water crisis that induced the 2008 cholera outbreak back to Harare's 'post-colonial water shortages and sanitation problems and the monumental errors of judgement by early colonial planners'.

Urban settlements in Zimbabwe were initially established as administrative and political structures for colonial rule. Early forms of urban structures were built on the bases of military settlements, camps and forts (for example, Fort Tuli, Fort Victoria, Fort Charter and Fort Salisbury) (Raftopoulos and Yoshikuni 1999). The first settlers of Salisbury constituted the so-called Pioneer Column. They had travelled from South Africa as part of the imperialist conquest of Cecil John Rhodes, the British mining magnate and governor of the Cape Colony. Rhodes's British South Africa Company endeavoured to find the 'Second Rand' – a new iteration of the Witwatersrand gold rush that led to the establishment of Johannesburg – from the ancient gold mines in Mashonaland. Staking their hopes on the possibility that a greater Witwatersrand lay under the sub-soil of Mashonaland, the township of Salisbury was initially planned as a frontier town for the habitation of 25,000 people with a 'commonage' of more than 20,000 acres encircling it (Yoshikuni 2007: 10). The frontier town was to be orientated toward racial separateness and economic exploitation. For Julie Seirlis, this movement demonstrated the militancy of Rhodesia's colonial expansion and its racial configuration of space:

> The topography of white spaces as a fortress, a citadel, a laager, is a profound expression of colonialism's militancy and a concrete expression of the politics of control and domination. It also emphasises the neurosis and paranoia built into the realisation of that control and domination because the fortress suggests a need for protection against a hostile environment, an attitude of defensiveness from a perceived or actual state of siege. (quoted in Raftopoulos and Yoshikuni 1999)

The drive for segregation in the frontier town was first entertained as a formal policy in 1892–93. Tsuneo Yoshikuni (2007: 28) recounts this history. He notes that the sanitary board considered removing 'all coloured people', including the Asians, to 'separate portions of the town'. In part, this was in response to a stream of Asian immigrants into Rhodesia's nascent urban areas. The idea was not a practical policy but a partisan expression of the ideal of 'total segregation'. By 1902, the Salisbury council adopted a similar position. The press mildly cautioned against this position, arguing that 'its feasibility or otherwise has yet to be determined'. Yet, in spite of the apparent impracticability of such a policy, the press proceeded to acclaim the proposal as a 'timely action' being 'in the best interests of the Municipality'. The salience of the council's position at this time was not the principle of total segregation itself, but the ideas invoked in its justification (Yoshikuni 2007). Central to these were claims of 'urban problems' such as the 'Black Peril' (the fear that black men would sexually prey upon white women) (McCulloch 2000) and the alleged public health problems, the 'sanitation syndrome' discussed below, caused by the presence of Africans in the city.

In this respect, the push for segregation was part of a wider trend in the region, which was just undergoing the process of capitalist, industrial urbanisation. In South Africa, segregated townships, called locations, were gaining official currency as a panacea for all manner of urban racial problems. For example, when the bubonic plague broke out in the port towns of the Cape Colony in 1901, serious attempts were made at expelling African workers from inner cities. During this time, urban race relations became widely conceived of and dealt with in the imagery of infection and epidemic disease. Maynard Swanson (1977: 410) calls this the 'sanitation syndrome' – the equation of black urban settlement, labour and living conditions with threats to public health and security – and he argues that it 'became fixed in the official mind, buttressed a desire to achieve positive social controls, and confirmed or rationalized white race prejudice with a popular imagery of medical menace'. This is amply illustrated by the racially selective application of quarantine regulations and disease control measures in Port Elizabeth during the bubonic plague epidemic of the early 1900s:

> Blacks were especially resentful at the discriminatory application of the plague quarantine regulations. Officials called it 'class discrimination', but their attitudes were clearly racial and Africans complained bitterly of maltreatment and abuse on grounds of colour. The houses of blacks had been quarantined; those of neighbouring whites had not. The possessions of blacks had been burned; the goods, the stores, and the warehouses where they worked and contracted the plague had not been touched, because those belonged to whites. (Swanson 1977: 402)

In essence, according to Swanson (1977: 387), the sanitation syndrome was a 'major strand in the creation of urban apartheid'. The Salisbury councillors were conversant with these developments 'down south' and sent letters to municipalities in the Cape Colony requesting information on urban locations (Yoshikuni 2007). The Cape government claimed to have relieved the city of 'its burden of uncivilized, low-paid, slum-bound, disease-ridden black labourers' (Swanson 1977: 394). This was, of course, merely a racist representation of Africans with no bearing on the actual epidemiology of infectious disease. Segregation was not driven by rational calculation, nor was it a universally accepted policy among the Rhodesians. This caused tension and disputes within and between government, industry and the communities, most notably between the settlers and the British South Africa Company, which ruled Southern Rhodesia from occupation in 1890–1923. The settlers accused the company of putting its own commercial interests ahead of settler social, political and economic preferences, which for many included total racial segregation (Mlambo 2014). To an important extent, it seems, Rhodesians were divided about how to provide for the mutual access of black labourers and white employers in the incipient industrial age without having to pay the heavy social costs of urbanisation or losing the dominance of Europeans over Africans.

The central state clashed with the Salisbury councillors over the extent of segregation in urban areas. The former downplayed the invective rhetoric of Black Peril or the 'sanitation syndrome' and instead insisted on greater liberties in housing and movement for African 'free' residents, that is, those Africans who were not 'accommodated' at their white employers' private residence (Yoshikuni 2007). To streamline the legislation regarding the locations, the Rhodesian government introduced the Native Urban Locations Ordinance (No. 4 of 1906) prohibiting African 'free' residence in Salisbury with full effect from 1 May 1908, and by the end of April 1908 the town police reported: 'all natives in the Township and on the Commonage, occupying premises, not used by their masters, have been warned they will have to remove to the Location on the 1st of May' (quoted in Yoshikuni 2007: 19).

During this same period, circa 1908, Salisbury underwent a 'municipal revolution' (Yoshikuni 2007: 11). With the failure to discover new reserves of gold in Mashonaland, the Rhodesian settlers shifted their focus to 'practical colonisation': extension of railways and roads; commencement of settler agriculture and land acquisition;

establishment of banks, mercantile houses and workshops; introduction of new transport facilities; institution of postal and other administrative services; and development of primary industries in areas like Hartley, Gatooma, Lomagundi and Marandellas (Yoshikuni 2007). The stimulation of business and economic growth fostered major civic improvements, perhaps the most outstanding of which was the introduction in 1913 of piped water and electricity supplies. In the process, Salisbury started to shed its hitherto militaristic outlook and assumed 'the more genteel trappings of a white middle-class paradise' (Seirlis 2004: 413). As settler colonialism took firmer root, Salisbury transformed for its white residents from a mere 'commercial and administrative centre' to 'a countrified suburbia where whites could live in the manner of landed gentry on mini-estates complete with rose gardens and servants' (Seirlis 2004: 414).

In October 1922, Britain held a referendum for Rhodesian settlers to determine their future either as part of the Union of South Africa, since the country was still formally ruled by the British South African Company, or as a self-governing entity. A majority vote passed in favour of the latter, making Southern Rhodesia a self-governing territory with a high degree of autonomy even though Britain retained control over foreign policy as well as the right to veto legislation seen as detrimental to Africans (Mlambo 2014). Successive self-government regimes entrenched segregation in the country through various measures to ensure African subservience (Mlambo 2014). The logic that ultimately prevailed – for the colonial state and the constituent classes of small businessmen, the railway establishment, white workers and city councils – was that urban space was a temporary place of work for Africans and was to be occupied so long as labour functions were being performed and at as little cost as possible to the central state and the city council. The authentic African locus of home and family in the settler colonial imagination was then recast as the rural area, the site of 'traditional' structures and control (Phiminister 1988; Raftopoulos and Yoshikuni 1999; Yoshikuni 2007; Ndlovu-Gatsheni 2009b; Musemwa 2012).

To take a panoramic view of the town, the growth of Salisbury generated a hierarchy of urban space. On a virtual sliding scale of residential prestige, the town transmogrified from the homogenous north-east, with its elegant, colonial-style bungalows and cottages, down towards the polyglot south-west, where an assorted collection of brothels, boarding houses, Indian shops, a Jewish synagogue, 'native locations', and the dwellings and stores of 'pioneers' were to be found (Yoshikuni 2007). The enforcement of segregation to protect the emerging 'white sanctuary' spawned a legislative labyrinth to control African movement into and within the city. For example, 'pass laws' were officially introduced under the Native Registration Act in 1936 to limit the African population's access to urban spaces while other laws imposed curfews on Africans; prohibited Africans from owning land designated as 'European'; and restricted African access to housing, typically provided for single male occupancy, thereby stemming the migration of rural families into the city (Phiminister 1988; Sapire and Beall 1995; Raftopoulos and Yoshikuni 1999; Yoshikuni 2007; Ndlovu-Gatsheni 2009b; Musemwa 2012).

Yoshikuni (2007) argues that the establishment of the urban location to house Africans must be seen primarily in the light of growing citizen pressure, especially emanating from working-class whites in the Kopje area of Salisbury, and not the 'sanitation syndrome'. He insists that there is little evidence to support the 'sanitation theory' often conveniently deployed by colonial officials to motivate their segregationist policy, and advanced by scholars like Lewis Gann and Peter Duignan (1970: 138–39), who argued that in Salisbury's early days 'there was no segregation ... In the 1900s, however, disease struck the shantytowns and convinced the white citizens that something must be done. They hastily cleared the infected area and shifted the Africans into a "location".' However, neither serious epidemic nor massive removals occurred at any point in the first decade of the twentieth century. The location policy focussed on clearing the town and was presented to white citizens as a solution to an imagined 'community crisis'. Underpinning the government's adoption and enforcement of racial segregation was a perceived rising threat of African economic competition, which was heightened during the austere economic times heralded by the Great Depression (Mlambo 2014).

The leading exponent of racial segregation was Godfrey Huggins, leader of the Reform Party, who assumed the role of prime minister of Southern Rhodesia from 1934 to 1953. Huggins advocated a 'Two Pyramid Policy', from 1938 onwards, of separate development for the Europeans and Africans. In his own words,

> The European in this country can be likened to an island of white in a sea of black, with the artisan and the tradesman forming the shores and the professional classes the highlands in the centre. Is the native to be allowed to erode away shores and gradually attack the highlands? To permit this would mean that the leaven of civilisation would be removed from the country, and the black man would inevitably revert to a barbarism worse than ever before .... Rightly or wrongly, the white man is in Africa and now, if only for the sake of the black man, he must remain there. The high standard of civilisation cannot be allowed to succumb. (cited in Mlambo 2014: 107)

The patterns and trajectory of urbanisation and segregated settlement were haphazard and disorganised despite efforts to generate a pristine 'white city' with a steady labour supply. These conflicts and dissonances are well documented by a range of scholars who have looked at the myriad ways in which Africans defied the intentions of discriminatory legislation and asserted their public presence within the city (see Raftopoulos and Yoshikuni 1999 for a summary).

Housing control was envisioned as a fundamental means, along with a pass and night curfew system, to control the behaviour and movement of the African worker. The colonial state and city council worked to confine African residence to either the employer-controlled servants' quarters or a municipality-supervised location. The housing estates provided at the latter were bitterly unpopular among Africans. Municipal involvement in African housing was the product of a demand for exclusion and the policy was characterised by 'utter disregard for the quality of tenants' lives' (Yoshikuni 2007: 41). Additionally, Yoshikuni argues, the council viewed the production of African housing in terms of revenue and, combined with housing controls, this enabled the council to charge a monopoly rate leading to a high rate of rent appropriation.

Another major strand of the council's involvement in the location was its preoccupation with social control. Further to the elaborate regulations governing the movement of Africans, the location was also placed under heavy police rule such that the townships were often enclosed within a barbed-wire fence and kept under surveillance. The high concentration of policing staff in very small locations augmented pressure on rents. Most importantly, the location was 'a bleak place', as Yoshikuni describes:

> Inside there existed no amenities, no schools, no shops, no churches and no clinics – only the large municipal beer canteen. In 1920 a neighbourhood of 250 huts shared just one borehole and three communal latrines, without a single ablution facility for them. (Yoshikuni 2007: 54)

At a general level, such regulations and measures of social control laid the foundations for the trajectory of housing in the townships.

Over time, overcrowding and inconsistency in the availability and quality of service provision have typified the townships. Another long-standing, major concern in the townships has been access to hygiene and sanitation facilities. From its very founding, the difficulty of acquiring sufficient supplies of water has persisted in the course of Harare's colonial and post-colonial history. In the late nineteenth century, prior to the 'municipal revolution', the colonial settlers sourced their potable water from springs, rooftops, individual wells and boreholes. And yet even with the provisions for piped water in Salisbury from about 1913, an amalgam of factors – such as climate; relief; geology and location on the central watershed (Tomlinson and Wurzel 1977 note the absence of sedimentary formations that could provide large aquifers in the vicinity of Harare); the long dry season with about eight months per year of minimum stream-flow; and the seasonal high rates of evapo-transpiration (Davies 1986) – all curtailed the city council's ability to secure reliable access to water as the city expanded.

Limitations on the water supply became a serious bone of contention in city council politics whenever the issue of latrine facilities for Africans was raised. In the early years of the colonial city, most business firms and private households failed to provide sanitary conveniences for their African workers. To address this, the sanitary board built a few 'native latrines' at street corners, but such facilities were totally inadequate for the needs of the African population. In 1895, the Township Sanitary Regulations (No. 109 of 1895) were introduced to compel every employer in Salisbury to provide latrines for servants. But the regulations had little influence on practice. Over time, as Salisbury gradually grew into an urban agglomeration, fears mounted about a potential infectious disease outbreak, such as typhoid or smallpox. Medical officials therefore repeatedly warned of the dangers of the dearth of sanitary facilities for the majority of the population, especially at a time when the town depended on wells for its water supply, but such alerts exerted minimal influence on policy decisions. Heated debates erupted at the town house but yielded no result, with the municipality often concluding that the cost of erecting 'native latrines' was too much for ratepayers (Yoshikuni 2007; Musemwa 2012).

The piped water distribution to the townships closely mapped onto the segregationist impulse and the prevailing assumption about African impermanence in urban areas. For the most part, the locations only received clean piped water, toilets and sewers as a fringe benefit of sanitary and water improvements occurring elsewhere in the city. Important predisposing, and mutually reinforcing, factors for the cholera outbreak thus obtained during this period. In 1953, Harare's current water supply system was laid down in parallel with the sewage disposal system, and both were situated in the same water catchment zone (Musemwa 2010). Additionally, the spatial pattern of topographical elevation in the city followed the socio-economic hierarchy of urban settlement whereby the low-density, affluent, white parts of the city were situated at higher altitude than the high-density, poor, African townships. Most of Harare was therefore located upstream of its main water supply. As such, the reticulation system depended on a sophisticated and elaborate hydraulic infrastructure of pumps and chemical treatment to deliver clean, potable water against the gravitational pressure gradient.[1] As a contingency plan against an engineering failure of the reticulation system, residents of the affluent areas of Harare had installed private boreholes to access groundwater directly and/or they were able to buy water from private sources that obtained water from outside the city. In the high-density townships, boreholes were extremely limited. Instead people dug shallow wells as an additional or alternative water source to the council water supply (Tomlinson and Wurzel 1977).

Given these observations, Musemwa (2012: 17) tentatively posits that 'with meagre sanitation amenities and rudimentary water technologies, the urban planners and administrators were setting up the townships as future sources of disease.' One key reason he offers for the lag time between the establishment of the townships and a major outbreak of diarrhoeal disease is Harare's relatively low rates of

[1] Interview, Peter Morris (water engineer), Harare, 7 January 2016.

Table 1.1 *Zimbabwe's urbanisation trends, 1961–2002*

Urban Centre	*1961–62*[a]	*1969*[a]	*1982*[a]	*1992*	*2002*
Harare	310,000	386,000	656,000	1,184,169	1,903,510
Bulawayo	211,000	245,000	414,000	621,742	676,787
Chitungwiza	–	15,000	172,000	274,000	323,260
Gweru	39,000	46,000	79,000	124,035	141,260
Mutare	43,000	46,000	70,000	131,367	170,106
Kwekwe	21,000	31,000	48,000	74,982	93,608
Kadoma	19,000	25,000	45,000	67,267	76,173
Masvingo	10,000	11,000	31,000	51,746	69,993
Chinhoyi	8,000	13,000	24,000	42,946	49,603
Redcliff	5,000	10,000	22,000	27,994	32,346
Marondera	7,000	11,000	20,000	39,384	52,283
Chegutu	7,000	9,000	20,000	30,122	42,959
Shurugwi	7,000	8,000	13,000	6,029	16,866
Kariba	6,000	4,000	12,000	21,039	24,210
Victoria Falls	2,000	4,000	8,000	15,010	31,519

[a] Estimates

Sources: Wekwete (1992); Government of Zimbabwe (2002); adapted from Mlambo (2014: 86).

urbanisation for much of its history because of the legislative control of African residence in the city under colonial rule. The percentage of urban-based African populations before 1978 had remained almost constant over the preceding seventeen years. However, as the liberation struggle for independence against colonial rule intensified in the 1970s, people in rural areas sought refuge in urban areas, resulting in a marked rise in the population of cities by 1979. With limited housing stock for Africans in the capital, overcrowding became inevitable in the locations. Salisbury's population expanded dramatically from 280,000 in 1969 to 633,000 by January 1980 (Patel 1984). Consequently, informal settlements proliferated within the townships on the periphery of the city. This process, described by Musemwa (2012: 18) as 'galloping urbanism' (see Table 1.1) exposed 'the insufficiency of the government's housing policy to satisfy the requirements of the urban poor for shelter and other attendant elementary amenities such as water, sewage, electricity and roads'.

Transforming Urban Order: The City and 'Modernising Development'

The liberation struggle for independence by African nationalist forces against Rhodesian rule lasted fifteen years, from the mid-1960s until the end of 1979. A bloody and destructive struggle, the war also saw the Rhodesian army using biological agents against the liberation movements. The techniques the Rhodesian forces used included poisoning wells; spreading cholera; infecting clothing used by insurgents; and killing cattle with anthrax to deplete insurgent food supplies, which resulted in the world's largest recorded anthrax outbreak (Martinez 2002). Rhodesia's Central Intelligence Organisation (CIO) and its special-forces regiment, the Selous Scouts, disseminated cholera in Mozambique and along the border to debilitate incursions from the eastern front. However, the CIO feared that the use of cholera could backfire and spread into Rhodesia uncontrolled and infect government army forces operating in the field. The use of cholera as a weapon was eventually discontinued because the agent was thought to dissipate too quickly to provide any lasting tactical advantage. Nevertheless, the use of cholera as a weapon in the liberation struggle would return to the fore of political consciousness and discourse over two decades later as I shall discuss in Chapter 3.

The conflict came to an end with the Lancaster House Conference in 1979 where an independence constitution, arrangements for the post-independence period and a cease-fire agreement were all put in place. Under these new arrangements, the country held elections in February 1980. The Zimbabwe African National Union, led by Robert Mugabe, now renamed ZANU-Patriotic Front or ZANU(PF), won an overwhelming majority with 57 seats in a parliament of 100 members. The other major nationalist movement turned political party, the Zimbabwe African Patriotic Union (ZAPU), garnered twenty seats, the United African National Council (UANC) claimed three seats and the Rhodesian Front took all twenty seats reserved for white Zimbabweans. The country formally marked its independence on 18 April 1980.

'As the sound of the celebrations died away after 18 April 1980, the sound of picks and shovels became audible; the *development* of Zimbabwe had begun,' wrote Nicholas Ndebele (cited in Auret 1990:

v, emphasis added), a former director of the Catholic Commission for Justice and Peace (CCJP) in Zimbabwe, when recalling the first decade of the country's independence from colonial rule. For the victors of the war, it was a period of hope and optimism as well as one of fierce ambition as ZANU(PF) endeavoured to transform the country and consolidate its political hegemony over its former colonial rulers and nationalist rivals. In concrete terms, the incoming government inherited an advanced manufacturing sector, sophisticated infrastructure, a relatively large network of banks and a highly technocratic, centralised and powerful bureaucratic state apparatus from its Rhodesian predecessor. As noted in the Introduction, the new ruling party, ZANU(PF), was quick to put this powerful machine to use in the service of 'modernising development' (Alexander 2010). Though technocratic and bureaucratic to a fault (Alexander 2010), the new government was able to deliver. Throughout the 1980s, the government expanded access to healthcare, education and sanitation. It initiated a large land resettlement programme in rural areas. The central legitimating claim of the new government was its promise to bring about development and modernisation (Karekwaivanene 2012). Crucially, the gains made in this period were not only material: they signalled the new government's aspirations to modernity, its capacity to deliver public goods as a source of political legitimacy, and its commitment to reversing some of the entrenched racial inequalities of the colonial period. Importantly, as Alexander and McGregor (2013) write, the government's capacity to deliver modernisation and development was facilitated, to a critical extent, by the commitment among civil servants to a professional ethic. This ethic was central to ZANU(PF)'s legitimacy and to civil servants' sense of self-worth.

For much of the 1980s, the ZANU(PF) government successfully capitalised on its success in the liberation war and its substantial victory in the independence elections. It was thus able to build a network of informal alliances with many of its former supporters and enemies (Dorman 2016). This coalition incorporated disparate elements such as white farmers, former Rhodesian politicians and Western donors. The 'politics of inclusion', to use Sara Rich Dorman's (2016: 33) phrase, became emblematic of ZANU(PF)'s early approach to nation- and party-building.

The post-independence government was nevertheless confronted with a series of choices and disputes as it attempted to reshape society and make a reality of its vision for the nation. Profound structural concerns such as post-war reconstruction and repurposing the inherited colonial political economy – especially redressing its racialised imbalances – existed alongside political challenges such as democratising the authoritarian colonial state and its institutions (Muzondidya 2009; Mlambo 2014; Dorman 2016). Equally difficult was the task of nation-building in a society with deep fissures along the lines of race, ethnicity, class, gender and geography. Such social divisions were compounded by the legacies of the liberation struggle on the country's political culture.

In this way, an uneven and contradictory picture of Zimbabwe's 'development' emerged in the 1980s. Dorman (2016: 45) notes that 'development' proved a compelling motivating force for government ideology – 'encapsulating all that had been denied by the Rhodesian regime'. In this the country received fervent support from a range of aid agencies and donors. The government implemented a policy of 'national development' that included the expansion and extension of public services to the black majority, especially in health and education, where it made notable achievements (Auret 1990; Muzondidya 2009; Mlambo 2014). The government expanded access to health facilities throughout most of the country: it restored 161 clinics that had been damaged during the war, built 163 new health centres and legislated free medical care for the poor. Regarding public health and preventative services, the government ran child immunisation schemes, nutrition and hygiene awareness campaigns, and family planning programmes. By 1990, Zimbabwe had the lowest child malnutrition rate in Africa as well as maternal and child mortality rates considerably lower than the continental average. The World Bank (1992: 7) cited Zimbabwe's achievements in health as 'truly impressive' in light of the above and other achievements.

Such accomplishments notwithstanding, James Muzondidya (2009: 169) characterises the gains made in the first decade of independence as 'limited, unsustainable and ephemerally welfarist in nature'. At a macro level, he contends that Zimbabwe continued to experience serious social and economic problems as well as redistributive challenges throughout the decade, especially in the spheres of land and the economy. Moreover, the economic boom of the immediate post-independence period was short-lived. At best, the economy experienced mixed fortunes during that time, as it went through the deleterious effects of droughts, weakening terms of trade, and high interest rates and oil prices. These factors diminished the state's capacity to finance its redistributive programmes.

Critiques of the Zimbabwean government's programme of 'development' can be taken further still. Gavin Williams (2003) reminds us that 'development is not a thing, it is an idea' – one whose polyvalent articulations give rise to overlapping, competing and contradictory politics, policies and programmes. In early post-colonial Zimbabwe, we see at least two radically different conceptions of development at play. On one hand, the new government presented 'the Zimbabwean people' as the drivers and beneficiaries of a nationwide and inclusive development project, especially as it sought to create distance between itself and the top–down development projects of the colonial era. As was en vogue in the late 1970s and early 1980s development discourse (Ferguson 1990), the new ruling party advocated a bottom–up and people-driven version of development (McGregor and Ranger 2000; see also Nustad 2001). The words of the newly inaugurated prime minister, Robert Mugabe (cited in Zimbabwe Government 1981), captured this sentiment best: 'Government is determined to embark on policies and programmes designed to involve fully in the development process the entire people, who are the beginning and end of society, the very asset of the country and the *raison d'être* of Government.' On the other hand, the ruling party, or elements within it, was also committed to its own vision of modernising development and orderliness.

Dorman (2016) sees the logics of coercive unity and top–down development as well as ZANU(PF)'s monolithic interpretations of citizenship – Shona-speaking, bearing totems, disciplined and making productive use of land – in both urban and rural areas. Additionally, a combination of the external threat from apartheid South Africa, persistent Cold War tensions and the strength of the inherited Rhodesian security state allowed for the continuation of a strong militaristic tendency by the ZANU(PF) government (Alexander, McGregor and Ranger 2000; Dorman 2016). Repressive legislation from the Rhodesian era was retained, along with an extended state of emergency (Mlambo 2014).

While my focus is on urban history, it is worth briefly mentioning how the ruling party dealt with significant challenges to its authority in rural areas in the 1980s, especially in the Midlands and Matabeleland provinces (largely Ndebele-speaking areas), in the form of ZAPU, its military wing and its civilian supporters.

The ceasefire of 21 December 1979 brought Zimbabwe's liberation war to an end. As already noted earlier in this chapter, this was a time of optimism but also one of ongoing insecurity and violence. Throughout the country, suspicious guerrillas from erstwhile antagonistic militaries and guerrilla movements had to turn themselves in to Assembly Points (APs), while long-secretive political cadres had to come into the open and order had to be consolidated to pave the way for elections. The loser in Zimbabwe's first national elections, ZAPU, soon found itself embroiled in political conflict, with devastating repercussions for its armed wing, the Zimbabwe People's Revolutionary Army, known as ZIPRA. Alexander, McGregor and Ranger (2000) offer a compelling and granular account of this period in their in-depth monograph, *Violence and Memory: One Hundred Years in the 'Dark Forests' of Matabeleland*. They note that partisan accounts of the post-independence conflict have portrayed it

> as the product of an ill-judged bid by ZAPU to claim the victory it had failed to gain through the ballot box, as a cynical attempt by ZANU(PF) to use the incidents of violence in the early 1980s as pretext to crush the only real obstacle to its total supremacy, or as an attempt by South Africa to exploit tensions between ZANU(PF) and ZAPU, whites and blacks, so as to leave its newly independent neighbour in disarray. (Alexander et al. 2000: 180)

As a challenge to such characterisations, these authors argue that post-independence insurgency was largely a result of distrust within, and then repression by, the newly formed Zimbabwe National Army (ZNA). During the liberation struggle, the two guerrilla armies' regional patterns of recruitment and operation had left ZIPRA forces dominated by Ndebele speakers from Matabeleland while the Zimbabwe National Liberation Army (ZANLA), the military wing of ZANU, was predominantly Shona speaking. Additionally, the guerrilla movement's operational areas maintained significance in terms of political loyalties: voting largely, though not completely, followed ethnic and regional divisions, creating the possibility for conflict along these lines after independence.

In brief, after the ceasefire, guerrillas were summoned to gather in designated APs from which they would be demobilised or integrated into the nascent ZNA. However, many guerrillas refused to come in to

APs and regularly cached arms and ammunition. While their motives were diverse, the most important was a pervasive fear that they would be bombed or attacked while concentrated in the APs, since the Rhodesian Army was, at this time, still very much intact. Internecine conflict soon ensued in the early 1980s within and beyond the ZNA involving newly formed state security forces, ex-combatants from both guerrilla movements, and civilians, who were drawn into the violence in complex ways.

In January 1983, Robert Mugabe's government launched a massive security clampdown in Matabeleland and parts of Midlands, led by a North Korean–trained division of the ZNA, known as the Fifth Brigade and itself a predominantly Shona-speaking formation (Catholic Commission for Justice and Peace in Zimbabwe 1997). Furthermore, this deployment coincided with the imposition of a strict curfew in the region. It soon became clear that the Fifth Brigade was not interested in seeking out 'dissident' soldiers from ZIPRA. Thousands of atrocities such as murders, mass physical torture and the burnings of property occurred in the weeks thereafter. Members of the unit declared to locals that they had been ordered to 'wipe out the people [Ndeble] in the area' and to 'kill anything that was human' (Alexander et al. 2000: 222).

The Fifth Brigade's motto was *Gukurahundi* (a ChiShona language term which loosely translates as 'the early rain which washes away the chaff before the spring rains'). Richard Werbner documents that peasants in Matabeleland said that they were the rubbish that the Shona wished to clear away (Werbner 1991). While the Fifth Brigade was active for a year, political and ethnic violence continued for much longer. The Zimbabwean human rights advocate and forensic anthropologist, Shari Eppel, estimates the total number of unarmed civilians who died throughout the entire *Gukurahundi* period to be 'no fewer than 10,000 and no more than 20,000' (cited in Cameron 2017). The precise figure remains uncertain. In addition to the killings, thousands more were arbitrarily arrested, detained without charge, beaten, tortured and raped, resulting in an intense atmosphere of fear and mistrust among the Ndebele.

The 1987 Unity Accord marked the end of the conflict and formally integrated the principal opposition party, ZAPU, into the ruling party under the existing moniker ZANU(PF). Authority was further centralised through the instatement of an Executive Presidency, held by

Robert Mugabe. The massacres foreshadowed a number of traits that would mark the authoritarian statism under the ruling party after 2000, namely the 'excesses of a strong state, itself in many ways a direct Rhodesian inheritance, and a particular interpretation of nationalism' (Alexander et al. 2000: 6).

In urban areas, Dorman points out that in the early 1980s, little changed with respect to the nature of the policies that were applied to governing the city, specifically the townships. Colonial era bylaws, plans and statutes largely remained in situ (Dorman 2015). There was an apparent tension between the imperative of overturning the racial and socio-economic segregation of Rhodesian city planning and that of maintaining a modern and orderly sense of urban space. In terms of housing, former 'white' suburbs in Harare were renamed 'low density neighbourhoods', and middle-class Black, Asian and Coloured families moved into them (Cumming 1993). Meanwhile urban high-density neighbourhoods expanded but few new suburbs were developed. Despite government plans in the early 1980s to build 115,000 units across the country, by 1985 only 13,500 were complete, and waiting lists grew longer and longer in the cities. With curbs lifted on racial segregation, the shortage of housing compelled impoverished urban arrivals to construct 'illegal' shelters in the townships.

In response, the government launched 'an almost unyielding battle against informal housing' from the 1980s onwards, and the antipathy of the Harare authorities to informal settlement, derisively called 'squatting', has 'remained a recurrent issue throughout the 1980s, 1990s, and into the twenty-first century' (Potts 2006a: 271). As such, the rational and modernising mission that had been espoused by the colonial state was retained, and 'squatting' was viewed by the new government as disruptive of this because it indicated improper land use and was seen as an encroachment on urban orderliness (Alexander 2006; Tendi 2010). In 1984, as reported by Potts and Mutambirwa (1991), there were eight 'squatter' settlements in Harare but forty-two others had been 'cleared'. Such processes showed little respect for the desperate urban poor who had resorted to 'squatting' out of economic necessity (Dorman 2016). Similarly, attempts were made to keep the central business district 'clean' and 'modern'. In striking continuity with colonial discourses, policies and practices, only formal businesses were supposed to operate in the city while informal markets and vendors were banned. In 1983, 'Operation Clean-up' was launched, and police arrested over 6,000 women in urban areas ostensibly to rid the streets of prostitution. In actuality, the arrested women included schoolgirls, women with babies and the elderly, many of whom were apprehended while commuting between work and home (Dorman 2016).

By the end of the 1980s, Deborah Potts (2006a) writes, it was evident that major contradictions and conflicts were arising between the needs of the urban poor and the desire and commitment of local urban authorities to maintain what they saw as an aesthetically pleasing and 'modern' urban environment, which conformed to planned land use schemes. The policing and eradication of illegal, 'squatter dwellings' was pursued with great vigour and to tremendous effect for most of the post-independence era. Thus, the government's efforts to maintain 'order' and a modern city image in Zimbabwe meant that the visual difference between Harare and most other major sub-Saharan African, let alone Asian or Latin American, cities in the 1980s and 1990s, and even into the early twenty-first century, was remarkable. While informal sector activities and begging were present on the street in the city centres, these were contained on a minor scale (Potts 2006a). No other African country, Potts observes, has maintained such continuity of official resistance to informal settlements (Potts 2006a: 284).

The 'galloping urbanism' of Harare at a population growth of over 5 per cent per year throughout the 1980s severely burdened the capacity of both central and local governments to provide accommodation and basic urban amenities for the urban poor (Musemwa 2012). From a water perspective, Harare's provisions had been relatively stable in the early 1980s. This was mainly because of the new Manyame Dam that had been built in 1976 to augment the city's water supplies (Musemwa 2006). Over the next ten to fifteen years and following the severe droughts of 1982–88 and much of the early 1990s, Harare, like other parts of the country, began to experience much more serious water shortages resulting from both ecological and political-economic factors.

The 'statist' economy of the 1980s may have succeeded in delivering many social welfare benefits to Zimbabweans while enjoying a growth rate of 4 per cent per year from 1986 to 1990 (Carmody and Taylor 2003), but it was not without its contradictions. An overvalued currency; arrears to international lenders; shortages of diverse essential goods such as paper, cement and vehicles; and the failure to adequately reduce pressures on land and achieve restitution in communal areas all contributed to the weakening of the national economy, the delivery of public services and ZANU(PF)'s political legitimacy (Muzondidya 2009; Alexander 2010; Mlambo 2014; Dorman 2016).

Under domestic and international pressure to address these political-economic conditions, the government implemented reforms in the form of an economic structural adjustment programme (ESAP). The ESAP package contained the standard features of IMF and World Bank economic reform strategies, including, *inter alia*: a reduction in the budget deficit through a combination of cuts in public enterprise deficits and rationalisation of public sector employment; devaluation of the local currency; trade liberalisation, including price decontrol, and deregulation of foreign trade, investment and production; phased removal of subsidies; and the introduction and enforcement of cost recovery measures in health and education sectors (Bijlmakers, Bassett and Sanders 1996). The latter sectors were badly affected by structural adjustment as evidenced by steep declines in key health and education indicators. Real per capita expenditure on health through the Ministry of Health and Child Welfare fluctuated dramatically in the 1990s, resulting in widespread difficulties in attracting and retaining qualified healthcare staff, the decreasing availability of drugs and medical equipment, the poor maintenance of buildings and the general decline in the quality of health services (Bijlmakers et al. 1996). From the patients' perspective, the introduction of cost recovery measures, specifically user fees, is thought to have profoundly altered health-seeking behaviour and diminished access to clinical care, especially among poor Zimbabweans, according to seminal studies at the time (Gibbon 1995; Bijlmakers et al. 1996, 1997).

The economic reforms of the 1990s led to a deterioration of urban living conditions through the expansion of the informal economy, as a consequence of unemployment and retrenchment, and the persistence of inadequate water and sanitation services. In high-density areas, exasperation with the delayed promise of development was amplified by the changes in living standards throughout the decade. At the end of the 1990s, it was evident that government policies would fail to meet their 1985 target of housing for all by the year 2000. In 1991, it was estimated that there was a deficit of 70,000 dwellings in Harare, based on the housing waiting list, which by 1994 had increased to

92,251 households (Dorman 2015). Homeowners responded to the demand for affordable housing, and their own declining incomes, by renting out rooms and backyard shacks to lodgers. Unable to spill over into vacant land, Harare's townships accommodated increasing numbers of people within limited space, resulting in more informal trade and worsening public health standards in terms of overcrowded housing and reduced access to clean water and sanitation facilities. Reactions to visible urban poverty were contradictory. Initially, as explained earlier in the chapter, the government had implemented 'clear-ups' and the forced removal of 'squatters'. From the 1980s to the 1990s, street-kids and the destitute were targeted for removal to holding camps, training centres and former refugee camps. However, as the 1990s wore on, tolerance of the informal economy seemed to increase. As Daniel Tevera and Amos Chimhowu's (1998) study of backyard shacks in Harare, concluded in the late 1990s,

> [T]he general mood has shifted from intolerance during the 'socialist era' of the 1980s to tolerance during the 1990s. The need to maintain a rapidly eroding political power base and to soften the impact of political hardships ... has compelled both central government and the Harare city council to grudgingly allow the proliferation of backyard shacks in the low-income residential areas.

The adoption of unpopular economic reform measures undermined the 'state expansion and social advance of the 1980s and, as a result, the government's ability to pursue its programme of modernising development' (Alexander 2010: 188). Additionally, the unbudgeted payouts to 'war veterans' through a pension fund in 1997 – to maintain their loyalty to the ruling party – as well as the tremendously high cost of involvement of the Zimbabwe government in the war in DRC in 1998 added to the failures of the structural adjustment programme by the end of the 1990s (Moore and Raftopoulos 2012). Furthermore, damaging allegations of corruption – most infamously the 'Willowgate' scandal in which several senior ministers were implicated in the illegal reselling of cars and trucks at much higher prices than they had paid (Dorman 2016) – diminished the popularity of ZANU(PF) in certain constituencies, for example in urban areas and among trade unionists, thereby helping to create space for the emergence of new forms of political opposition through the decade. This culminated in the formation of the Movement for Democratic Change (MDC) in

1999, a new political party that forged an alliance among a diverse coalition of interests and that presented ZANU(PF) with its first serious electoral challenger since independence in 1980. The ensuing confrontation between the two parties ushered in a period of political disruption and economic upheaval with profound consequence for public service delivery, urban infrastructures and political order.

Disrupting Urban Order: The City and the Crisis

The 2000s witnessed a major urban crisis in Zimbabwe. Manifest as a series of resource-based emergencies, such as fuel, food and electricity shortages, this crisis was rooted in the country's economic meltdown and political conflicts (Ranger 2007; Raftopoulos 2009; J. L. Jones 2010b; Chiumbu and Musemwa 2012; Dorman 2015). As Raftopoulos (2009: 201–02) explains,

> This upheaval consisted of a combination of political and economic decline that, while it had its origins in the long-term structural economic and political legacies of colonial rule as well as the political legacies of African nationalist politics, exploded onto the scene in the face of a major threat to the political future of the ruling party, ZANU(PF). The crisis became manifest in multiple ways: confrontations over the land and property rights; contestations over the history and meanings of nationalism and citizenship; the emergence of critical civil society groupings campaigning around trade union, human rights and constitutional questions; the restructuring of the state in more authoritarian forms; the broader pan-African and anti-imperialist meanings of the struggles in Zimbabwe; the cultural representations of the crisis in Zimbabwean literature; and the central role of Robert Mugabe.

In the years leading up to the cholera outbreak, the ruling party deployed an array of legal, coercive and patronage strategies to transform state bodies from bureaucratic to partisan institutions (Kamete 2006; Ranger 2007; Muchaparara Musemwa 2008a; Alexander and McGregor 2013; McGregor 2013). Terence Ranger (2007) describes how the ZANU(PF) government, especially since 2000, dismissed elected executive mayors; sacked whole municipal councils; and appointed partisan commissions to run the cities. The Combined Harare Residents' Association (CHRA) – an umbrella community-based organisation that aims to represent and support all residents of

Harare by advocating for effective, transparent and affordable municipal and other services – identified the Urban Councils Act as integral to ZANU(PF)'s strategies for seizing greater control of local government:

> On the one hand it bestows a degree of local autonomy to residents through local council elections, yet on the other it confers almost dictatorial power upon the Minister of Local Government ... This legislative confusion has given rise to the serious conflict that has undermined the good governance of the capital city. (cited in Ranger 2007: 161)

ZANU(PF)'s actions were triggered by its defeat at the polls in urban areas from 2000 onwards. In February 2000, the ruling party supported a new constitution, which was decided upon in a national referendum. The proposal was unexpectedly defeated and was taken as both a personal rebuff for President Robert Mugabe and a political triumph for the newly formed opposition. In June, Harare's electorate, like their urban counterparts across the country, rejected ZANU(PF)'s bid to represent them in parliament (Kamete 2006). All nineteen constituencies elected opposition MDC Members of Parliament. Subsequently, in the council and mayoral polls of March 2002, the electorate again voted against ZANU(PF) candidates thereby stripping the ruling party of all vestiges of democratic representation in the capital. And in the simultaneous presidential polls, Harare voted overwhelmingly in favour of Morgan Tsvangirai. To all intents and purposes, ZANU(PF) had become 'a rural party'. The defeats of 2000 spurred ZANU(PF) into action, and the party sought to reassert its dominance in urban politics – to re-urbanise, as it were. In the process of trying to regain urban control, ZANU(PF) turned urban governance into the object of intense political struggle, and drastically undermined the capacity of councils to deliver services. The ruling party's strategy hinged on recentralising powers over local authorities, developing a system of patronage through and beyond local state institutions, creating 'parallel' party hierarchies and using party-aligned militia to control key urban spaces and access to resources (McGregor 2013).

An integral element of the ruling party's strategy was the 'reassertion' of formal planning, which resonated with people's memories of past (both colonial and post-colonial) enforcement of urban regulations, limitations on informal markets, and sometimes evictions and clearances (Fontein 2009). Potts (2006b: 291) explains the overarching motivations of the 'slum clearances' and demolition exercises that followed as threefold:

> a desire to punish the urban areas for their almost universal tendency since 2000 to vote for the opposition MDC; an ideological adherence to modernist planning and the associated image of a 'modern' city; and a desire to decrease the presence of the poorest urban people, by driving them out of the towns, because of an incapacity to provide sufficient and affordable food and fuel for them.

The most notorious 'clearance' was launched on 19 May 2005, when Sekesai Makwavarara, chair of the government-appointed and unelected Harare Commission that was running the city, announced that the City of Harare intended to embark on Operation *Murambatsvina* (meaning 'Restore Order' or 'Drive Out the Rubbish'), a programme to

> enforce by-laws to stop all forms of illegal activities. These violations of the by-laws in areas of vending, traffic control, illegal structures, touting/abuse by rank marshals, street life/prostitution, vandalism of property infrastructure, stock theft, illegal cultivation among others have led to the deterioration of standards thus negatively affecting the image of the City. The attitude of the members of the public as well as some City officials has led to a point whereby Harare has lost its glow. We are determined to bring it back ... It is not a once-off exercise but a sustained one that will see to the clean-up of Harare ... Operation Murambatsvina is going to be a massive exercise in the CBD [Central Business District] and the suburbs which will see to the demolition of all illegal structures and removal of all activities at undesignated areas. (cited in Potts 2006a)

What followed, dubbed by many as 'Zimbabwe's tsunami', was a massive campaign – unprecedented in scale and duration throughout the history of urban Africa, including in apartheid South Africa – of forced evictions from 'illegally squatted' areas as well as bulldozers flattening informal markets and homes, offering owners and inhabitants only minutes to remove property (Potts 2006b; Fontein 2009). This was especially so in high-density areas across Harare and other cities. The most authoritative report, written by Anna Tibaijuka (2005), the UN Special Envoy on Human Settlement Issues in Zimbabwe, conservatively estimated that around 650,000–700,000 people had lost either their homes or the basis of their livelihoods, or often both, during the operation. These findings were derived from the government's own estimates and average household size, and information gathered from a range of different organisations and individuals within the country.

Despite official pronouncements about the need to 'restore order' – to reassert formal planning procedures, bylaws and local state institutions – Operation *Murambatsvina* was experienced as the arbitrary, extreme and often violent execution of state power by council officials, police and the military, which for many seemed to operate outside the bounds of a legitimate and bureaucratic authority (Fontein 2009). Enforcing the sense of sinister intent behind the demolition and clearances exercises, Police Commissioner Augustine Chihuri reportedly said that the purpose of the operation was 'to clean the country of the crawling mass of maggots bent on destroying the economy' (cited in Tibaijuka 2005). In my own interviews with township residents, the operation still evokes painful memories of being assaulted by the state and plunged into homelessness, destitution and 'suffering.' Even just mentioning it stirred difficult emotions for Paida, resident in Norton, 'Murambatsvina. You're making me think. Sometimes, you mustn't think about that because you will hate life.'[2] Moreover, if the aim was to restore Harare's 'sunshine' status, *Murambatsvina* often created more squalor than it removed (Fontein 2009). In many cases, good-quality housing was destroyed, only to be replaced by ramshackle, temporary structures – previously a rare sight in Zimbabwe even if characteristic of so many informal urban settlements across the continent. And, notably, many township residents blamed Operation *Murambatsvina* for creating the conditions that allowed cholera to spread in urban areas: '[T]hey are partially to blame for that cholera. That outbreak occurred soon after *Murambatsvina*, so there was dilapidation of infrastructure. Even here there was a toilet outside and it was destroyed. It worsened the outbreak.'[3]

Conclusion

In this chapter, I have provided a focussed history of Harare's urban environment and the fraught politics of orderliness, social control, development and disruption that have shaped it. Through my

[2] Interview, Paida, Harare, 31 October 2015.
[3] Interview, Favor, Budiriro, 23 September 2015.

discussion of how national and local governments have, at different points in history, intruded into the economic and social life of township residents, two salient themes for the study of the politics of cholera are apparent. First, the problems of urban overcrowding and the difficulties of delivering public services, including water and sanitation, to high-density areas are enduring, and they predisposed Harare's townships to diarrhoeal disease outbreaks. These patterns were neither arbitrary nor accidental, but were the outcomes of strategies of social control, political repression, myopic urban planning and racist ideas of African impermanence in the city. Second, in the post-colonial period, the formal extension of civil and political rights to township residents was not sufficiently accompanied by improvements in social and economic conditions. The townships have remained an ambiguous space of inclusion and exclusion. Urban residents have enjoyed greater freedoms in the city through the lifting of pass laws and segregation, but they have also been subjected to projects of formal 'planning' and the 'reassertion' of order, such as demolition exercises, which have resulted in dispossession and displacement. As will become even clearer in the next chapter, it was the urban poor who were most affected by Zimbabwe's rapidly declining basic public services as well as by the urban planning and 'order' to which official justifications of Operation *Murambatsvina* appealed (Fontein 2009).

This chapter has also discussed ZANU(PF)'s angry reaction to what it saw as illegitimate challenges to its authority. The ruling party fought back on multiple fronts, using legal, militaristic and patronage strategies to take over state institutions, manipulate elections, discredit and undermine the opposition, and reassert its presence in urban areas. These changes had profound ramifications for state institutions and social services. The next chapter examines these changes more forensically through a two-stage analysis: a dissection of how the post-2000 crisis precipitated the cholera outbreak; and an examination of how the outbreak unfolded and which factors perpetuated its spread.

2 'When People Eat Shit'

Cholera and the Collapse of Zimbabwe's Public Health Infrastructure

When you look at cholera, it's not a health issue. It only happens when people eat shit.

—Portia Manangazira, Interview, Harare, 2015

In this chapter, I explain how an easily preventable and eminently treatable disease became such a massive calamity thereby throwing the failure of Zimbabwe's public service delivery systems into sharp and detailed relief. In the preceding chapter, I delineated the structural factors that predisposed Harare's townships to a diarrhoeal disease outbreak. Central to my argument was the claim that historically embedded social inequality laid down the underlying physical conditions – namely poor sanitation facilities, inadequate clean water provision and overcrowded housing – for the potential spread of an epidemic in the high-density areas of the city. This chapter presents the institutional and infrastructural factors that precipitated the outbreak and that perpetuated its spread in 2008–09.

Attention to infrastructure is as crucial here as it was in the last chapter. In all my discussions with officials in the ministries of finance, health and local government; with development experts in the WHO, UNICEF and the IOM; and with aid workers in numerous international NGOs, I was repeatedly told that the cholera outbreak was a crisis of 'health infrastructure'. In conversation and reports, public health experts talked about Zimbabwe's 'dilapidated system in terms of piping and infrastructure'.[1] They explained that 'the major causal factor' of the cholera outbreak 'was the dilapidated infrastructure, the sub-standard infrastructure'.[2] They reported that cholera had compounded the 'implosion of the health system and basic infrastructure'

[1] Interview, Oxfam Water and Sanitation Specialist, Harare, 8 September 2015.
[2] Interview, Steven Maphosa, WHO Environmental Health Officer, Harare, 24 September 2015.

(Médecins Sans Frontières 2009a). Therefore, this chapter takes infrastructure seriously and discusses what Alice Street (2014: 2) refers to as 'the sheer materiality of health system architecture'. This 'sheer materiality' powerfully informs the stories and political subjectivities that I discuss in Chapters 3, 4 and 5.

I argue that the origins, scale and impact of the cholera outbreak were overdetermined by a multi-level failure of Zimbabwe's public health infrastructure. I situate this multi-level failure in the country's political conflicts and economic crisis, which created a 'perfect storm' for the fulmination of cholera. My argument draws inspiration from the historian, Charles Rosenberg. As I explained in the Introduction, Rosenberg (1992) argues that two predominant modes of analysis have been deployed to explain epidemics: contamination and configuration. The notion of contamination is strongly associated with diarrhoeal diseases, as these infections are transmitted by the passing of morbid material from one person to another. However, Rosenberg warns us that such a style of analysis is reductive and mono-causal; it fails to recognise the interaction of the myriad environmental factors necessary for the successful transmission of infected material between persons. Instead, Rosenberg advocates a 'configurational' style of explanation wherein epidemics are understood as a consequence of a unique convergence of material and social circumstances, in this case the collapse of the healthcare delivery system, the multi-level failure of the water reticulation system and the political economy of daily life. However, I go further than the concept of 'configuration'. I argue that the cholera outbreak gives us a clear view of the changes that ZANU(PF) wrought in Zimbabwe's state institutions and practices in key sectors such as healthcare delivery, provision of water and sanitation, ensuring pubic access to food and the regulation of informal trade.

The chapter is organised around three principal features of Zimbabwe's health infrastructure. First, I discuss how the most immediate causal factor for the severity of the epidemic appeared to be the dysfunction of the healthcare delivery system. Cholera was able to disseminate through the country without an effective system to detect it, to disrupt its spread or to provide timely treatment to its victims. But as Dr Portia Manangazira, the former deputy and now current Director of Disease Control and Epidemiology in the Ministry of Health in Zimbabwe, pointed out to me, '[W]hen you look at cholera, it's not a health issue. It only happens when people eat shit.'[3] Put differently, despite the moribund state of Zimbabwe's healthcare delivery system in 2008, the primary determinants of the cholera outbreak were situated in the wider set of forces and systems shaping the material conditions of daily life and in the collapse of infrastructure needed to deliver essential resources.

As I explained in the Introduction, cholera requires 'a very gross level of contamination, greater than for any other known epidemic disease', to produce illness in normal individuals (Carpenter 1976), and therefore it only tends to appear in epidemic form in contexts where sanitary conditions are poor; where malnutrition is widespread and severe; and where people are living in overcrowded housing or temporary settlements. Thus, the second major factor that I examine was the spectacular mismanagement and sabotage of Harare's water reticulation system – a critical factor in precipitating and perpetuating the outbreak. The third factor I look at relates to the livelihood changes ushered in by Zimbabwe's disastrous economic downturn. These changes, referred to here as the political economy of daily life, rendered vast swathes of the population vulnerable to cholera through food insecurity and malnutrition. Additionally, the expansion of informal trade networks during this period facilitated the adventitious spread of the disease.

Finally, it is worth mentioning that the cholera outbreak provoked multiple and contested debates within and beyond Zimbabwe about why it occurred. These debates are given their due attention in subsequent chapters. In what follows, I offer my own analysis of the multiple linkages between the collapse of public service delivery and the origins, scale and impact of the cholera outbreak. I draw upon interviews with officials in the ministries of finance, health and local government; with development experts in the WHO, UNICEF and the IOM; and with aid workers in numerous international NGOs. I combine these discussions with documentary sources such as reports and post hoc evaluations of the outbreak from government bureaucracies, UN agencies and NGO reports. Many accounts of the outbreak are intertwined with interpretations, judgements and claims about why it happened. Inevitably, I note some of these in passing here but I analyse them fully later in the book.

[3] Interview, Portia Manangazira, Harare, 9 September 2015.

A Total Health System Collapse

I spoke at length to Professor Margaret Borok, Head of Internal Medicine at the University of Zimbabwe Medical School, about working conditions in the national health system over the last two decades. As Borok sees it, the decline in Zimbabwe's hospital services was incipient in the 1990s during the structural adjustment era, as discussed in Chapter 1. The HIV/AIDS epidemic devastated the health sector further. In terms of scale, HIV prevalence in women attending antenatal clinics in Harare increased nearly fourfold between 1989 and 1994, rising from 10 per cent to 36 per cent. By 1999, 1.5 million people of Zimbabwe's total population of 11 million were estimated to be infected by the virus. Of those infected, 1.4 million were aged between 15 and 49 years, representing approximately 25 per cent of the most economically active age cohort – thus Zimbabwe had the second most extensive AIDS epidemic in the world after Botswana (UNAIDS/WHO 2000). By 2006, AIDS was reportedly killing 2,500 people every week (Mlambo 2014). The health system suffered a double hit from AIDS: on one hand, it was overstretched by the high prevalence of the disease in the general population, while on the other, there were high infection rates among healthcare workers, including doctors and nurses, severely enfeebling the delivery of medical treatment.

This deterioration proceeded apace with the onset of the crisis in the early 2000s before plummeting to its nadir in 2008. Borok recalls 2008 with immense frustration and anguish:

> In the hospital, it was things like drug supplies. You wanted to do a test but there were no reagents for basic things like blood counts, electrolytes. It slowly got worse and worse. The x-ray machines weren't working. The radiotherapy department wasn't working. There was no chemotherapy unless you bought it privately. My [Kaposi's Sarcoma] patients just didn't get it or if they did it was vastly overpriced. Those kinds of things were very distressing to work with because we watched people dying. That's really hard. People in renal failure weren't being dialysed. There wasn't a catheter. Those are hard things to watch. You try to teach students about what they should be doing but that's a hard thing to do. I can talk to someone about conservative management of chronic renal disease but on the ground with a patient in front of you ... that's a hard thing. A lot was to do with supplies; some was to do with training, the conditions of service were shocking

because there was no buying power. I think it was in 2008 and everybody was given $100 (per month) across the board and that was the government's solution to try and retain staff. In fact, I think it was called a retention allowance. In retrospect that's just outrageous in terms of the level of people that it was aimed for. That's pitiable, if we're going to be honest about it.[4]

Indeed, the health system was *in extremis*. Clinical coverage was inadequate throughout much of the country, forcing patients to travel long distances for treatment. At medical facilities, there were critical shortages of essential medicines while frequent electricity outages prevented the use of much hospital machinery. Basic equipment such as disposable gloves, syringes, rehydration fluids and bandages were in desperately short supply, leaving patients and family caregivers to purchase these items elsewhere.[5] Staff were underpaid or not paid at all for months on end. Those with the resources, connections or opportunities set up private clinics or opted to work for international organisations, leading to a profound hollowing out of the national healthcare system.[6] Government and donor white papers (Chikanda 2005; Dieleman, Watson and Sisimayi 2012) reported that Zimbabwe had witnessed a veritable exodus of skilled health workers, especially from the public sector. In December 2008, per the government's official and likely conservative estimates, owing to the difficulties of accurate data capture, the public-sector vacancies in the health sector were at 'unacceptable levels of 69% for doctors, 61% for environmental health technicians, over 80% for midwives, 62% for nursing tutors, over 63% for medical school lecturers and over 50% for pharmacy, radiology and laboratory personnel' (Government of Zimbabwe: Ministry of Health & Child Welfare 2013: 9). Of the staff still working, the majority were unmotivated and inexperienced. Few had ever seen a case of cholera before and even fewer knew how to set up a cholera treatment centre.[7]

From Portia Manangazira's perspective, the Ministry of Health and Child Welfare had difficulty encouraging Zimbabweans in different parts of the country to attend national health centres when they became ill: '[T]he population had lost confidence in our system. They

[4] Interview, Margaret Borok, Harare, 5 October 2015.

[5] Interview, Stanley Midzi (WHO/Ministry of Health), Harare, 22 September 2015; Portia Manangazira, 2015 int.

[6] Interview, Dr Frances Lovemore, 6 October 2015.

[7] Portia Manangazira 2015 int.; Stanley Midzi 2015 int.

had gone to the clinics many times and they would be lucky to get paracetamol, or one of the simpler antibiotics, the rest of the stuff was just out of stock.'[8] For instance, I spoke to an elderly woman, a survivor of cholera, in the high-density township of Budiriro who put it like this, 'Imagine you are sick, you go to the clinic and there is no medication. You are just going to die. There was no money for treatment.'[9] Paida, a thirty-three-year-old woman living in Norton, echoed this exasperation when relaying to me the death of her infant, 'If you go to the clinic, sometimes no doctors, no treatment. No one to attend to the child. And he died.'[10] Furthermore, both women observed that most people resisted going to the clinics until the last possible minute. Deterred by a tragic combination of fear and denial, the urgency of feeding children at home and the unattractive prospect of staying in overcrowded, underserviced, dilapidated facilities, many township residents did not seek treatment until they were left with no other choice.

In the context of the country's astronomical hyperinflation, Manangazira noted that 'you would order [medical supplies] for $10 million [Zimbabwe dollars] but in 3 days when the signatures are being sought, it's already $25 million [Zimbabwe dollars] and how do you approve? It was just that kind of a scenario.' Further to this already extensive catalogue of difficulties, the health system lacked the necessary surveillance capabilities – including testing laboratories, technicians and chemical reagents – to track and report emerging epidemics in a timely manner.[11] For these reasons, Manangazira observed that, ironically, the health system itself had become a structural driver of the cholera outbreak. Manangazira relayed to me that in her ministry's post hoc evaluations they acknowledged the health system as a 'determinant' of the cholera outbreak. It lacked the staff: '[I]f you do not have the bodies – this is a service industry – who is going to treat the patients? Who is going to screen them and triage? That's very important in emergencies.'[12] It lacked the stuff: 'We had a huge shortage. We lost some cases because we didn't have enough IV fluids to resuscitate these cases. Cholera cases, normally they lose fluids very rapidly through vomiting and diarrhoea. You need to replace them quickly.'[13]

[8] Portia Manangazira 2015 int. [9] Elderly woman in Budiriro 2015 int.
[10] Patience 2015 int. [11] Margaret Borok 2015 int.
[12] Portia Manangazira 2015 int. [13] Stanley Midzi 2015 int.

The space was unsafe: 'People were being mismanaged. The infection control practices were not quite there. Most people did not know how to set up a cholera treatment centre so that you minimise spread and maximise the care and management of the patient.'[14] The communication and transport systems were compromised: '[T]hose [surveillance] systems were not working because the phone was cut off ... the transport system was not working either ... You then have things happening in the community and we have no idea that they are happening.'[15] And as Paul Farmer has famously argued, in public health and healthcare delivery, without staff, stuff, space and systems, nothing can be done (Farmer et al. 2013).

At a press teleconference in the middle of the cholera outbreak, Dr Christophe Fournier, the International Council President of Médecins Sans Frontières (MSF), made this very point emphatically:

> I have just returned from visiting our teams in Zimbabwe to assess our medical programs. What I witnessed in the last few days is the kind of health crisis that we as MSF doctors usually only see in war zones, or in countries in the immediate aftermath of conflict. Zimbabwe is a country literally falling apart at the seams. But beyond the cholera epidemic is a total health system collapse. Cholera is the tip of the iceberg. Health facilities are closed and patients simply cannot access health care. Medical staff has fled because they are not paid; there is an acute shortage of essential medicines and medical materials; and in those few places where services are still available, patients cannot afford care as they have to pay in foreign exchange. (cited in Médecins Sans Frontières 2009d)

In addition to the structural challenges discussed above, the ZANU(PF) government politicised the cholera outbreak in harmful ways. I discuss this at length in the next chapter. Here I highlight some of the most important disputes between different institutions of government, which undermined the cholera response. Through the Ministry of Information, the government initially denied the presence of a cholera outbreak, thereby preventing civil servants in the Ministry of Health from calling upon a desperately needed full-scale international emergency relief apparatus. To quote a medical doctor and health activist from a local NGO who spoke to me about the confusion around the emergence of cholera, the suppression of information and the collapse of the health system,

[14] Portia Manangazira 2015 int. [15] ibid.

While the cholera was starting, there was all this stuff going on with diamonds. There were rumours of cholera and then Beatrice Infectious Disease Hospital became a no-go zone. They were trying to suppress information. I think it took about six or seven weeks before they actually started documenting the deaths correctly. It took quite a long time. You have to remember that nobody was going to work. The other thing that you need to know was that at both Harare Hospital and [Parirenyatwa] Hospital, the doors were padlocked. Nobody was going to work because nobody could find enough money to pay the transport to get to work. The whole medical system was dysfunctional. Everybody was aware that cholera may become a problem but nobody really wanted to talk about it, including the international community who were very hesitant about putting any more fuel on the fire of this burning Zimbabwe. ... The military blocked the information. It was a good six weeks before we started getting any type of epidemiological reporting. ... and the state just didn't want the UN agencies in anywhere. They really didn't want anyone to see the mess they made. ... The big issue was that it was one crisis too many. And no one wanted to admit that actually, everything had failed.[16]

Additionally, through both the military and provincial governments, the ruling party restricted humanitarian access to several parts of the country to prevent aid workers and journalists from broadcasting the extent of devastation caused by the disease.[17] MSF provided a nuanced commentary on the response of the government to the crisis, noting the ways in which different state institutions engaged with outside assistance:

Zimbabwe's response to the humanitarian crisis varies from one ministry to the next. MSF has had a positive working relationship with the Ministry of Health, treating many cholera patients in Ministry of Health structures alongside the ministry's own staff. At the other end of the scale, the authorities have blocked MSF's attempts to respond to the broader, less visible components of the health crisis. Despite glaring humanitarian needs, the government continues to exert rigid control over aid organisations. (Fournier and Whittall 2009).

Portia Manangazira articulated the double bind of delivering healthcare during cholera outbreak in a politically divided environment as follows:

[16] Interview, Activist, Harare, 6 October 2015.
[17] Interview, Brian Patrick, Aid Worker, London, 6 July 2015.

> Our job is to prevent secondary cases arising, prevent mortality, prevent complications, manage the outbreak, and tell the president that we have done enough and that we are seeing a reduction in the number of cases, it is no longer increasing but we still have a situation. As a technical people, we still have that mandate whether or not the politicians are supporting us ... the politicians' mandate is to improve their popularity and whatever they say may be in tandem with that; but in terms of us, we are supposed to look at what the international guidelines are – what WHO advises regarding outbreak detection, management and control. This is why you have health workers working in a crisis situation.

Beyond the 'total health system collapse' that I have described, cholera was also a symptom of an epic failure of Zimbabwe's water reticulation systems, especially in urban areas. I discuss this below.

Troubled Waters

Urban water supply became a crucial site of struggle for control between ZANU(PF)-aligned state institutions and municipalities run by the opposition MDC during the post-2000 crisis. An important juncture came in 1998 when, in an ostensible attempt to rectify the colonial imbalances in water supply, especially in urban areas as discussed in Chapter 1, and to mitigate against the risk of severe droughts as happened in the early 1990s, the government rewrote the Water Act (Youde 2010). The stated goal of the new act was to improve the water delivery infrastructure and to enhance equity of access to water. To this end, the new Act began by designating water as a public, rather than private, resource. The government established the Zimbabwe National Water Authority (ZINWA) in 2000 as 'a wholly Government owned entity tasked with managing the country's water resources' with a mandate to 'sustainably deliver quality water to all our communities (Rural and Urban) whilst making strategic water infrastructure investments that facilitate human and economic development' (ZINWA 2011). At its founding, ZINWA took over the development and management of national water resources and the associated infrastructure throughout the country except for Harare and Bulawayo (Youde 2010). By May 2005, ZINWA had been given jurisdiction in Harare as well. ZINWA charged fees for water supply to cover the costs associated with providing water. In theory, these reforms 'should have provided more people with access to water while also providing the funding necessary to maintain and improve the water infrastructure' (Youde 2010: 696).

From the outset, however, ZINWA was an instrument of President Mugabe's 'political machinations' (Youde 2010: 696). As part of ZANU(PF)'s strategy to rebuild its urban electoral support in Harare, the party saw water provision as an important means of controlling an essential function of local government, of demonstrating its legitimacy through service delivery and of undermining the MDC by diminishing the opposition's role in governing (Musemwa 2008a; Youde 2010). Furthermore, the creation of ZINWA facilitated the siphoning of funds away from water and sanitation to military and security forces loyal to the ruling party (Bratton 2014). In the course of my fieldwork, I failed to interview anyone who could speak with authority and candour about the inner workings of ZINWA through the 2000s. I am thus unable to offer new empirical insights into how and why the organisation was used to serve partisan ends. Whatever the case, the organisation failed to achieve its water-related reforms. Instead of bolstering the country's water infrastructure and improving access, the creation of ZINWA actually decreased water access substantially and caused the near-collapse of the water reticulation system (Youde 2010). In 1988, 84 per cent of Zimbabweans had reliable access to safe drinking water; in 2008, over 70 per cent of Zimbabweans lacked such access, with Harare losing 40 per cent of its water supply every day due to burst pipes and leakages (Musemwa 2008a).

The view that ZANU(PF) nationalised the water for financial gain was echoed to me by several people in different social and professional arenas – including public health and water specialists in development organisations, Zimbabwean water engineers, residents in Harare's high-density areas and urban activists from the Combined Harare Residents Association and the Water Alliance. These views are captured by a Zimbabwean aid worker at the International Rescue Committee:

> [B]efore 2008, most [city] councils were now from opposition parties, there were not so many people from the ruling party that were in council. I would think it was a political move just to take away that responsibility. And also, City of Harare relies on water for its revenue, mainly. I remember that soon after that move, City of Harare was then struggling – struggling! – to pay workers. Struggling even to provide some of the services that they could

provide before the water was [nationalized] ... so now all the money was going to [politicians via ZINWA], City of Harare didn't have anything.[18]

This perspective accords with the literature on Zimbabwe's urban crisis. Joost Fontein (2008), Muchaparara Musemwa (2008b; 2010), Boniface Coutinho (2010), Jeremy Youde (2010) and Michael Bratton (2014) all argue that the creation of ZINWA deprived the local councils of an important source of revenue and severely crippled their capacity to deliver public services. ZINWA had acquired the water and sanitation infrastructure in Harare without providing any compensation to local government authorities. In one fell swoop, years of capital investment were lost. In Harare, the technical and financial implications of ZINWA taking control of the water supply were devastating: a lack of accountability, an inefficient and pliable bureaucracy largely controlled by the ruling party, internal struggles and general hostility toward MDC-aligned institutions of local government (Musemwa 2010; see also McGregor 2013). As exemplified by ZINWA, the politicisation of state institutions meant that there was little scope for professional practice: an official expelled by the government-appointed commission to run Harare in lieu of the mayoral office, then later reinstated, said, 'We are technocrats and the councillors are politicians – that is how it is supposed to be; they make policy and we advise from a professional point of view. But when officials are also politicians, where is the space for professional judgement?' (cited in McGregor 2013).

As Harare was afflicted by perennial water shortages, ZINWA lacked the technical, human and financial resources to supply water, to fix waterworks when pipes burst, and to dispose of sewage safely. Peter Morris, a Zimbabwe-based civil engineer who was involved in the water-systems response to the cholera outbreak through UNICEF, German Agro-Action and the Zimbabwean government, helped to conduct the most widespread analysis of the failure of the country's water reticulation and supply processes. He explained to me how the urban water crisis helped to precipitate the epidemic.[19] Morris asserts that a critical shortcoming of ZINWA was the inexperience of its staff. Prior to assuming control of almost all of Zimbabwe's water supply

[18] Interview, Aid Worker, International Rescue Committee, Harare, 18 September 2015.

[19] Interview, Peter Morris, Harare, 7 January 2016.

systems, the most complex system that ZINWA had managed was in the 'tiny' jurisdiction of Karoi – a town in the North of the country with a population of approximately 25,000 people. In Karoi, ZINWA was 'responsible for the treatment and the distribution [of water] within the low-density and commercial areas and the local authority was responsible for the distribution to the high-density areas'.[20] It was therefore a major leap to go from managing water supply in the small jurisdiction of Karoi to managing the byzantine water reticulation system of Harare. Further still, the country's hyperinflation severely compounded ZINWA's problems:

> There were also problems of working in a hyperinflationary environment. When you read the [water] meters, and get the bills out, it's going to be probably at least a month from the time when you read the meter to when you get paid or maybe longer. And if the value of the money is halving every month or every week, you're on a highway to nothing. You'll never get the revenue you need to run the city. Any utility runs on money. It's cash flow. If you don't have the money to run it then you can't run it. … Hyperinflation was really important. And it was a management issue. ZINWA was not capable of managing systems.[21]

A combination of long-term structural factors such as the siting of the water supply system in the same water catchment zone as the sewage system, the poor maintenance of the contemporary water system since it was first established in 1953 and the misalignment of water provision to population needs; political choices such as the nationalisation of water under ZINWA; and the economic crisis particularly hyperinflation all contributed to the material collapse of the water system's infrastructure. This collapse can be understood in three broad categories: (1) phenomena associated with hydrodynamic changes; (2) phenomena associated with vessels and their vicinity; and (3) phenomena associated with contamination of the water flowing through the system. I discuss each of these categories in turn.

Phenomena Associated with Hydrodynamic Changes

The primary problem was not the quality of the water but the mechanics of water treatment and delivery. An effective reticulation system

[20] ibid. [21] ibid.

depends on the turbulent flow of water. Hydrodynamic changes, such as stasis with interrupted flow, result in a plethora of problems. Firstly, all pipes in a water system will develop a biofilm. A biofilm is a group of microorganisms in which cells stick to each other, and often these cells adhere to a surface, in this case the internal lining of a pipe. While this is a process that occurs in all water systems, the formation, development and character of the biofilm depends on the physico-chemical properties of the water flowing through the system. In Zimbabwe, the water is replete with naturally occurring organic matter such as the remains of organisms, plants and animals, and their waste products. These organics provide fertile terrain for the growth of bacteria and fungi, and this manifests as an especially thick biofilm. In a continuously pressurised system, the biofilm stabilises itself and strongly adheres to the surface.

In Harare, most of the city is located upstream of its main water supply. As such, the reticulation system depends on a sophisticated and elaborate infrastructure of pumps and chemical treatment to deliver clean, potable water against the gravitational pressure gradient. In 2008, every water treatment plant and pumping station in the country was functioning poorly and was thus unable to provide continuous water pressure through the system. The interrupted flow – extended periods of stasis followed by upsurges of turbulent flow – disturbed the natural lining of the pipes. In this way, the biofilm contaminated the luminal water flow, resulting in the discharge of black and green water from domestic and industrial pipes. While no investigation was done at the time, it is plausible, even likely, that the biofilm contained cholera *vibrios*, among its many microbes, during the outbreak.

Phenomena Associated with Vessels and Their Vicinity

Another issue closely related to the intermittent supply of water was the leaking of the vessels carrying water and the contamination of groundwater in the vicinity of the pipes. The leaking of pipes is unavoidable in any water reticulation system, as Peter Morris explained to me: 'Even in Germany [pipes] leak. So, while the system is pressurised, your safe water inside the pipes is going out into the soil and the water that's in the soil will go back into the pipes.' Under normal circumstances, this is usually not a problem. Where there is turbulent flow, the degree of contamination is often too low to be

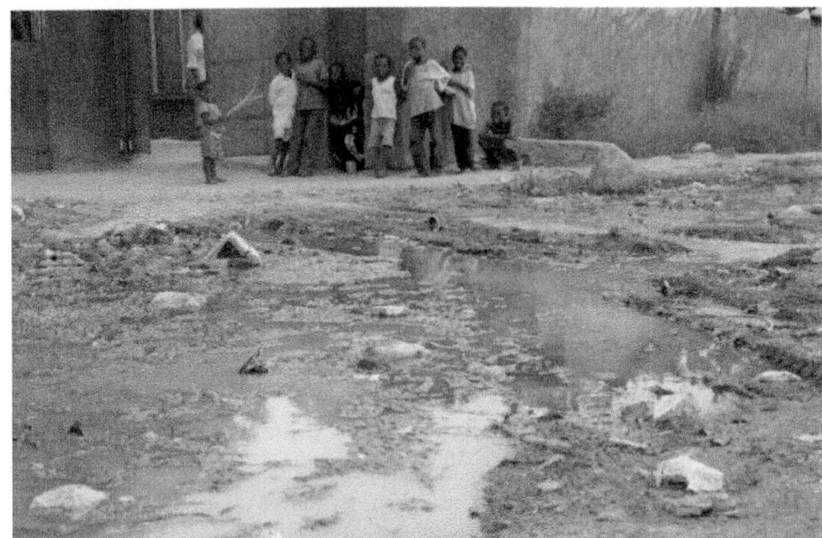

Figure 2.1 Raw sewage spills onto a street from a burst sewer main in the high-density suburb of Chitungwiza on the outskirts of Harare.
Source: Jason Tanner Photography.

consequential so long as the pressure is sustained and the quality of the pipes is maintained. Additionally, as water, typically from rain or irrigation, permeates the soil to reach groundwater, it is subjected to natural filtration through physical, chemical and biological processes that remove or degrade various constituents within it.

In Zimbabwe, the pipes were leaking at an inordinately high rate because they were old, had not been kept in good repair, and were liable to burst. The same was true of the sewage system. The subterranean sewage pipes were seeping large volumes of human waste into the groundwater, which flowed into the water delivery system because of the leaking pipes and the proximity of the two systems. Above ground, burst pipes and open sewers spilled raw sewage onto the streets of the high-density townships such as Chitungwiza and Budiriro (see Figure 2.1). Accordingly, the water available to township residents was contaminated below ground when sewage seeped into the piped water supply, and it was contaminated above ground when free-flowing sewage and other waste was washed by rain, down the sloping gradient of the city, into the shallow wells that were commonly used as a water source in lieu of council water (Luque Fernandez et al. 2012).

Phenomena Associated with Contamination of the Water Flowing through the System

In Zimbabwe, most of the water that enters the reticulation system is initially drawn from a dam. It then goes through a standard treatment process. In the first stage, a flocculant (a chemical that removes suspended solids from liquids), typically aluminium sulphate, is added to the water to coagulate the impurities in the water and allow them to settle. The water is then transferred to a settlement tank, where it is filtered and chlorinated with necessary adjustments made to the pH (level of acidity or basicity) of the water. In Harare, the process is much more complicated because of the physico-chemical properties of the water that comes from the Manyame dam, the city's main water supply. In this case, the water treatment process includes, inter alia, the addition of acid, activated charcoal and a sodium silicate flocculant aid. Once the water has been so treated, it is then pumped into reservoirs – Harare's main reservoir is Lake Chivero – where it is stored before being delivered into the network that distributes the water to homes and places of work for use and consumption.

During the crisis, these processes failed at every step. Owing to hyperinflation, embezzlement and underinvestment, ZINWA could not purchase the required chemicals needed at treatment centres, like Morton Jaffray Works, Harare's principal treatment plant. Combined with the failure of pumping mechanisms, this led to perennial water shortages in Harare and other cities throughout the 2000s. The Integrated Regional Information Network (2008b) reported that at one stage in 2008, ZINWA was so desperate to deliver some water into the reticulation system that it bypassed the initial treatment processes and began 'pumping raw sewage into Harare's water supply dam, Lake Chivero'. As such, the water coming out of the taps often emitted a pungent smell and contained green algae from the lake.

What I have shown in this section is the multi-level failure of Zimbabwe's urban water reticulation system. In complex systems, such as this, catastrophe rarely results from single-point failures, but rather from a multitude of weaknesses throughout the system (see Cook 1998). In other words, each of the individual failures that I have highlighted was necessary to cause catastrophe, but only the combination of them was sufficient to cause an overall breakdown of the system.

The Political Economy of Daily Life

As initially explained in Chapter 1, the post-2000 crisis resulted in dramatic changes in livelihoods for much of the population. The instability of money was a central feature of the changes afoot. Not only was the Zimbabwe dollar being liquidated; so too were the middle- and working-class lifestyles that had been built on the currency (Jones 2010a). It is estimated that during this period less then 20 per cent of adults were in formal employment (Chiumbu and Musemwa 2012). Formal-sector wages and salaried labour were replaced by relentless and uncertain efforts to 'get by' (Jones 2010b). The very notion of price lost almost all correspondence with any conception of 'fairness'. Indeed, as Jeremy Jones (2010a) writes, it was difficult to know what was fair; prices for goods depended immensely on time, place and individual relationships. The absurdity of the country's hyperinflation is illustrated by the outlandish changes in price of even the most basic items:

> On 1 August 2008, an egg in Harare, Zimbabwe, cost five Zimbabwe dollars (ZWD, widely referred to as Zimdollars). By February 2009, when the Zimdollar was replaced by legal trade in foreign currency (GOZ 2009), the same egg cost two trillion Zimdollars – a 40 trillion percent increase in the space of six months. (Jones 2010a)

The government attempted to 'discipline' hyperinflation by imposing a complex regime of price controls, accompanied by the unremitting printing of money. This, however, only resulted in further and more frequent shortages of consumer goods as producers claimed costs of production were not being met (Jones 2010a). Jones (2010a) points out that for most people, basic goods could only be sourced from the so-called 'black market'. The dynamics of this market are too intricate to summarise here. What is crucial to note is that basic goods were subject to price controls – a practice that dates back to the pre-independence era, which was then, after a brief suspension in the 1990s, revived in 2001 (Jones 2010a). As local production declined precipitously after 2000, every attempt the government made to enforce controls only led to the complete disappearance of controlled goods from the formal market, until such a time as enforcement waned. Making matters worse, those with access to goods at official prices – for instance, state employees and ZANU(PF) leaders – could accrue large profits by channelling goods to a desperate black market, where prices were much higher.

By 2007, on the rare occasions when cooking oil or sugar was delivered to a local retailer, it would quickly be purchased by dealers who would then resell a large portion of it on the black market (Jones 2010a). As a result, Jones (2010b) and Musoni (2010) argue that Zimbabwe experienced a profound 'informalisation' of its urban economies, and people became primarily oriented towards short-term rewards and survival. Most of the population turned to informal trade and bartering, engaging in heterogeneous activities such as vegetable vending and illegal foreign currency trading as well as pilfering at work and bribe-taking. Much of the skilled artisan production force emigrated, primarily to Botswana and South Africa, where they often engaged in unskilled labour, trivial commerce or cross-border trade (Jones 2010a, 2010b; Musoni 2010).

At the same time, urban politics remained fraught with intense power struggles between the ruling party and its main opposition culminating in one of ZANU(PF)'s most spectacular measures to assert its authority and re-establish its presence in urban areas – Operation *Murambatsvina*. The operation, discussed in the previous chapter, tied into the bigger economic crisis adding homelessness, squalor and further infrastructural damage in the townships to food, fuel and currency shortages (Dorman 2015). These different dimensions of the crisis rendered day-to-day life nearly impossible. An immediate consequence of the crisis were widespread, critical food shortages that triggered a sharp rise in acute malnutrition, especially among the poor and the vulnerable (Hove-Musekwa et al. 2011). Waste management, not only of sewage but also of household refuse, had effectively ceased to be done by government authorities and was instead improvised by individuals and communities. Harare-based epidemiologist and public health specialist, Rene Loewenson, closely tracked these developments and made the following observations:

> I think that there were a lot of problems with food security because of the unavailability of food and the cost of food . . . It was really becoming difficult

for ordinary people to access decent food. People were getting food in all kinds of informal ways. And then waste management was extremely poor. The local authorities had serious problems with being able to manage even the most basic of the public health obligations that they had. Things were just happening in an *ad hoc* and informal way. People were dumping waste, some people were burning things, people were dumping them in sanitary lanes, and so on and so forth. I would say that there was a real breakdown in many dimensions of public health. And I think the authorities that were charged with responsibility to deal with this, that had the duties – whether from ministry or from the district – were in a financial crisis as well. … Ordinary people were just preoccupied with staying alive and doing whatever they could and the authorities were preoccupied with just dealing with the financial crisis and so on. And people were letting things happen. I think that was very much the kind of environment within which you find that epidemics break out.[22]

I spoke to residents of the Dzivarasekwa township who described the abject need for food in their communities, especially since *Murambatsvina* but reaching its lowest point in 2008: 'We learnt to cook mangoes and paw-paws. We were eating a wild root that is normally eaten by horses and donkeys.'[23] In the rural areas, the situation was just as dire if not worse, as families were 'surviving on wild berries or nuts that they grind into powder and mix with water, a weed called lude that they boil into a thin soup. They also eat insects such as locusts … Some even eat the moist inner fibres of bark' (cited in Ndlovu 2012: 117).

The shortage of food in the country was so severe that more than two million Zimbabweans relied on food assistance to survive by the end of 2008. The United Nations Food and Agricultural Organization predicted that the figure would rise to 5.1 million in 2009 (45 per cent of the population) (cited in Sollom 2009). The distribution of food relief was primarily focussed on rural areas, rather than cities, and was intensely politicised. Physicians for Human Rights (PHR), an international human rights NGO, conducted a covert investigation into health and human rights in Zimbabwe towards the end of 2008. The organisation reported that the army prevented supplies of maize meal from 'being delivered to many in Matabeleland and other rural areas, such as Binga and other parts of the Midlands, that had voted against

22 Inteview, Rene Loewenson, Harare, 14 November 2015.
23 Focus group discussion, Dzivarasekwa, 7 October 2015.

Mugabe' (Sollom 2009: 26) in 2008. The same report charged that the state-owned Grain Marketing Board sold inexpensive maize, but officials would sell the grain only to card-carrying members of the ruling party while those suspected of supporting the opposition were denied access to food. Furthermore, the government restricted the operations of aid organizations, such as Save the Children and Oxfam, thereby preventing large quantities of food from being distributed.[24] In June 2008, the Minister of Public Service, Labour and Social Welfare, Nicholas Goche, announced that the government had banned 'all humanitarian NGOs from operating in the country' (Sibanda and Zhangazha 2008). In a circular to the NGOs, Goche said:

> It has come to my attention that a number of NGOs involved in humanitarian operations are breaching the terms and conditions of their registration as enshrined in the Private Voluntary Organisations (PVO) Act (Chapter 17:05), as well as the provisions of the Code of procedures for the Registration and operations of Non-Governmental Organisations in Zimbabwe (General Notice 99 of 2007). ... As the regulatory authority, before proceeding with the provision of Section (10) sub-Section (c) of the Private Voluntary Organisations Act (Chapter 17:05), I hereby instruct all PVOs/ NGOs to suspend all field operations until further notice. (cited in Sibanda and Zhangazha 2008)

It is difficult to assess how many people died from starvation and malnutrition from about 2007 to 2009, as there are no comprehensive or reliable data available. What is certain is that acute malnutrition and hunger induced greater susceptibility to cholera in the population and exacerbated its pathological effects in those affected. As epidemiologists and medical anthropologists have demonstrated, the co-existence of two or more diseases may synergistically interact to produce a higher degree of pathogenesis (an example would be HIV and tuberculosis co-infection). Referred to as 'syndemics', these mutually reinforcing processes suggest a biosocial model that conceives of disease in terms of its interrelationships with pernicious social conditions and interactions, and thus as a distinct expression of mass suffering; 'it would make us more alert, as well, to the likelihood of multiple, interacting deleterious conditions among populations produced by the structural violence of social inequality' (Singer and Clair 2003: 434). In this case, cholera was

[24] Interview, Oxfam, Harare, 8 September 2015.

synergistically linked with malnutrition, caused by high levels of food insecurity across the country:

> Malnutrition and cholera are intensely interconnected as cholera remains a disease of the world's poorest people. People who are malnourished are more likely to develop cholera infection, and cholera is more likely to flourish in places where malnutrition is common, such as refugee camps, impoverished countries, and areas devastated by famine, war or natural disasters. Poor nutritional status results from many causes such as limited food availability, poor nutrient intake, depressed appetite, malabsorption and metabolic disturbances. . . . In 2008–2009, Zimbabwe experienced a sharp rise in acute child malnutrition leading to a worsening cholera epidemic. (Hove-Musekwa et al. 2011)

The Perfect Storm

Act I

Zimbabwe's 2008–09 outbreak was not the country's first. The first major cholera outbreak in recent years was in 1993 in which the WHO reported 5,385 cases and 332 deaths from the waterborne disease. In 1998, a localised outbreak resulted in 335 cases of cholera and 12 deaths. Six years later, cholera claimed 40 lives and caused 900 illnesses. And in March 2006, yet another cholera outbreak killed 27 people (IRIN 2008a). According to Dr Stanley Midzi – former Director of Disease Control and Epidemiology in the Ministry of Health and Child Welfare (2005–09) and current Health Systems Strengthening Officer at the WHO headquarters in Harare – Zimbabwe started experiencing periodic cholera outbreaks around 1972 during the war for liberation.[25] Midzi explains that outbreaks of the disease would appear about every ten years and usually 'in the periphery districts, particularly those which are bordering Mozambique'. An assessment by the WHO's Global Task Force on Cholera Control (2006) confirm that the disease is endemic in the Manica province of Mozambique, which borders eastern Zimbabwe. From the late 1980s and through the 1990s, the epidemic cycle shortened to every five years. In terms of disease prevention, reductions

[25] Interview, Stanley Midzi, Harare, 22 September 2015.

in national hygiene promotion programmes in the wake of structural adjustment (Bijlmakers, Bassett and Sanders 1996), droughts and crop failures, and the poor maintenance of public health infrastructure such as water and sanitation, are among the factors that account for the changing patterns of the epidemic (Echenberg 2011). During this time, rural areas were affected far more than cities. Nevertheless, Midzi argues, there was still adequate sanitation coverage through much of the country to protect the overwhelming majority of local populations and communities and to rehydrate affected cholera sufferers either at home or in clinics. As importantly, the health system was responsive. It had a robust early warning system and reacted promptly to signs of a nascent epidemic through early treatment of confirmed cases followed by contact tracing and targeted hygiene promotion campaigns in the relevant areas.

From 2000 onwards, however, Midzi posits that Zimbabwe's political-economic crisis increased the frequency of diarrhoeal disease outbreaks. He reports that the Ministry of Health picked up suspected or confirmed cases of cholera on a yearly basis. He argues that the fast-track land reform programme compelled large numbers of people to migrate to areas 'where the sanitation coverage was not meeting the corresponding demand ... there was a dilution of coverage down to less than 24% for sanitation and less than 50% for water coverage' exposing more people to low-quality or untreated water. Additionally, water shortages meant that township residents could not use indoor toilets leading to open defecation outdoors or use of pit latrines. At the same time, many people relied on water fetched from shallow wells, which exposed them to bacteria via surface runoff or contamination from nearby pit latrines.

Underfunded, the capacity of the healthcare system to prevent or respond to cases of acute watery diarrhoea was diminished. In 2006, the Zimbabwe Association of Doctors for Human Rights (2009; see also Youde 2010) in conjunction with other local health organisations warned the government of a 'cholera time-bomb' if immediate action was not taken to improve health services and repair the water and sanitation infrastructures. Trudy Stevenson, an MP for Harare north (2000–08) and a founding member of the MDC, proposed a motion in parliament for the 'restoration of democratic local government' on 8 February 2006. In her statement she raised the alarm about a cholera outbreak on the horizon in the capital city:

[W]e have reports of cholera, we have health warnings being given out by the City of Harare workers themselves that there is a danger of cholera in Harare. We have the Association of Zimbabwe Doctors for Human Rights releasing statements about two weeks ago, highlighting the outbreak of cholera and highlighting the danger of further outbreaks of disease in Harare and elsewhere, if we do not do something about our service provision, which is what we are supposed to do. (Hansard, Parliament of Zimbabwe, Wednesday 8 February 2006: cited in Zimbabwe Association of Doctors for Human Rights 2009)

Further still, Portia Manangazira, explained that among the 'tell-tale signs' of an impending cholera outbreak was the marked increase of the 'diarrhoea caseload' that her department had been attending to, especially since 2006. But, she notes, what was not anticipated was the potential magnitude of a cholera outbreak; moreover, the ministry had underestimated the incapacitation of both the preventive and responsive arms of the public health system. Steven Maphosa, an environmental and public health officer who worked for the Ministry of Health for eighteen years before joining the WHO in 2003, remarked that the cholera outbreak was eminently predictable:

We in fact saw it coming because over the years, especially when I was in the Ministry of Health, we had what is called a National Taskforce of Epidemic-Prone Diseases when all provinces came, local authorities came, and we were debating and discussing on the various health problems in the areas around the country. And one prominent thing that featured was the poor water and sanitation infrastructure in urban areas. At that time, Harare was a nightmare, it had flooded so much [with sewage from burst sewer pipes]. In olden times, infrastructure was done for a very small population but now it had gone so old and needing replacement. We were always discussing about it but eventually this happened.[26]

Act II

By 2008–09, the proverbial time bomb exploded with cataclysmic effect. Politically, the country was in turmoil following heavily disputed presidential elections in the first half of 2008. Elections were initially held at the end of March with mediation from the Southern Africa Development Community and they proceeded with relatively

[26] Interview, Steven Maphosa, Harare, 24 September 2015.

little violence. However, following a delay of five weeks in the release of the electoral results, it became evident that, for the first time in its twenty-eight years in government, ZANU(PF) had blatantly lost its parliamentary majority. The combined MDC won 109 seats compared to ZANU(PF)'s 97. Controversially, the presidential contest between three candidates – ZANU(PF)'s Robert Mugabe, the MDC's Morgan Tsvangirai and former Minister of Finance, Simba Makoni, running independently – failed to deliver a decisive winner with a '50 per cent plus one' majority. Tsvangirai polled at 47.9 per cent of the vote while Mugabe won 43.2 per cent, thereby requiring a run-off election. Brian Raftopoulos (2009) argues that ZANU(PF)'s loss was a result both of the party's internal divisions and its growing loss of legitimacy amongst the electorate, in the context of the country's economic collapse. The defection of Simba Makoni, once a party stalwart, to stand as an independent presidential candidate demonstrated the fissures in the ruling party.

In the interregnum between the March elections and the presidential run-off at the end of June the country was plunged into further political uncertainty, marked by the worst violence seen in the country since *Gukurahundi* (Alexander and Chitofiri 2010). Under the instruction of the Joint Operations Command of the armed forces, the violence was mostly carried out in the three Mashonaland provinces, former strongholds of ZANU(PF), and targeted at MDC supporters and at ZANU(PF) supporters who had not voted for Mugabe in the presidential poll. Violence also erupted in urban areas, including in the high-density townships, opposition strongholds, that were soon to become epicentres of the cholera outbreak. Below, I share an excerpt of a conversation I had with Paida and her mother, Maria, to give a sense of the internecine violence that gripped the townships:

MARIA: The people hate the government. So that's why president says soldiers are now allowed to beat people. There were too many soldiers beating people. I was beaten by soldiers in Dzivarasekwa. I was beaten! I have a mark.

PAIDA: 2008, that's when we had elections. There was a lot of violence then! A lot! The people were beaten, my friend! The youth, boys and girls, were taken to the base. Just imagine a girl taken to the base. The whole night there.

SC: And what did they do there?

PAIDA: Ah obvious! Obvious! For the boys, if it's ZANU(PF) and they just suspect that you are MDC, they take you to the base. They torture you there. Some people were burnt. Burnt. Some to death. Or they take a metal rod that is red hot and put it right round the body. That base, it was near our house about 200 metres away.

MARIA: Youth from MDC, they are making petrol bombs. And when they know that someone is ZANU(PF), they would throw the bombs at them.

PAIDA: Ah, it was otherwise. During the elections, people were beaten. People were beaten. Even if you support ZANU(PF), you mustn't show people that I am supporting ZANU(PF). If you support MDC, you mustn't show people that you support MDC. You keep that in your heart. If they saw it, you pay for it.[27]

Faced with such widespread violence, Tsvangirai withdrew from the run-off, giving Mugabe a de facto solo but ultimately pyrrhic 'victory'. Mugabe's electoral success was met with a universal lack of recognition leaving Zimbabwe without a legitimate government in the eyes of the 'international community' or indeed from the perspective of the majority of the electorate (Raftopoulos 2009).

All the while that this was happening, the overlapping crises of the collapsed health system, the multi-level failure of the water reticulation system, and the political economy of daily life converged to create a 'perfect storm' for a ruinous cholera outbreak. As Renee Loewenson articulated it,

> [F]or me, the situation is that when you get this coincidence between informal population movement and an inability of the local governance arrangements to service that population movement especially in urban areas but also rural and you've got a massive movement of waste, and informal markets, and collapse of urban water supply and sanitation, and no trust between the people and local government, then whatever the political context you're in, you're at high risk of an outbreak whether it be cholera or typhoid or another type of epidemic.[28]

Comparing a range of technical reports as well as interviews with several doctors, epidemiologists, public health specialists and aid

[27] Interview, Maria and Paida, Harare, 31 October 2015.
[28] Renee Loewenson 2015 int.

workers, the precise beginning of the cholera outbreak is impossible to determine. While the Ministry of Health and the WHO's official report on the joint response to the cholera outbreak (2013) cites the beginning of the outbreak as August 2008,[29] several other sources suggest that the initial cases occurred much earlier but, for a range of technical and political reasons, were not reported.[30] Crucial in this regard was the relative absence of governmental medical and public health entities on the ground to respond to the country's deteriorating humanitarian crisis. The recording of the start of the outbreak was further complicated by the ban on almost all the international relief organisations working in the country. Ajay Paul, an aid worker with German Agro-Action – one of the few international organisations operating in Zimbabwe throughout 2008 – gave me an anecdotal account of the start of the outbreak, which offers insight into the multitude of technical and political problems facing the health system at that time:

> The outbreak started ... the first reported cases came from Binga but they were not verified by the Ministry of Health. The timeliness of the response for an outbreak like this is absolutely key. With the Ministry of Health structure for reporting – usually going from district to provincial to national level then the sharing and dissemination of that information is, in the case of notifiable disease like cholera, not fit for purpose. It doesn't do the job, it doesn't allow you to respond. We're talking about really remote rural locations in Binga, places like Manjolo, Nyami Nyami, and there was also a reluctance by the Ministry of Health to accept that there had been an outbreak for many reasons. Your interest is in the socio-political dynamic at play in the country at that point and there wasn't a great deal of enthusiasm to broadcast a situation that progressively was deteriorating.[31]

In Stanley Midzi's account, the most senior technocrats in the Ministry of Health first learned of a cholera outbreak while they were attending a national malaria conference at a holiday resort in Kariba in August 2008: 'When we came back [to Harare] ... we found out that the number of cases were actually much more than what we expected and what we received ... the surveillance system was not sensitive enough

[29] Triangulated with interviews from Stanley Midzi (WHO/Ministry of Health), Portia Manangazira (Ministry of Health), Steven Maphosa (WHO/Ministry of Health) and Goldberg Mangwadu (Ministry of Health).

[30] Multiple interviews with humanitarian aid workers.

[31] Interview, Ajay Paul, German Agro Action, Harare, 8 October 2015.

to pick the correct picture.'[32] Not only were the early cases not picked up accurately, thereby denying the health authorities of the state and the humanitarian sector a true assessment of the epidemic, but the disease began to spread with uncontained ferocity. As Ajay Paul put it,

> Traditionally the outbreaks in Zimbabwe of cholera have been in rural areas. We haven't seen cholera in urban areas. Of course, with people moving around and the mobility factor coming into play, you can have urban cases but the index case usually originated in rural areas in Zimbabwe. Mid-August ... we had the first reports from Chitungwiza ... The outbreak spread from there really really fast. It was then in Budiriro and then in Chinhoyi and then in Kadoma and then just all across the Mashonalands in particular. The scale obviously caught everybody off guard. All agencies were behind the curve. We were all behind the curve. We were always chasing it. We needed to take much quicker action with chlorination of urban supplies, large-scale; getting point-of-use disinfection out there; there weren't enough partners with experience in health to be able to do that. WHO systems were just totally unprepared and unable to cope. You had a volatile mix: you had an epidemic that was spreading fast in rural areas and in [densely] populated [urban] areas; you had public health services that were on the verge of breakdown because doctors and nurses were on strike; you had the lack of capacity, and partners and resources, to do simple interventions like setting up ORS [oral rehydration solution] points and other key life-saving interventions, not enough partners knew how to do that; we had clinics, primary health clinics, that were completely overwhelmed.[33]

Act III

The first officially confirmed cases were reported in August 2008, with eleven deaths by September. The Norwegian government responded quickly with US$7 million for water treatment but this did not halt the disease's seemingly inexorable spread. The distribution of cholera cases followed an identifiable spatial pattern related to the active population movements and densely populated areas, as shown by Luque Fernández et al.'s (2011: 7) ecological study:[34]

[32] Stanley Midzi 2015 int. [33] Ajay Paul 2015 int.

[34] Ecological studies are studies of risk-modifying factors on health or other outcomes based on populations defined either geographically or temporally. Both risk-modifying factors and outcomes are averaged for the populations in

Southern suburbs of Harare have numerous bus stops, where people from Chitungwiza arrive in the city for work. Often adjacent to these bus stops are crowded informal markets, popular with commuters, with very poor sanitary conditions. Our results show that the mobile working population (15–44 years of age) represented the greatest proportion of cases, strongly suggesting that the combination of a highly mobile infectious working population coming together in the overcrowded and unsanitary conditions found in markets significantly influenced the spread of cholera into the city through person to person transmission.

Over the next three months, the government refused to designate the outbreak as either a 'state of emergency' or 'national disaster'. This would have allowed the UN agencies to activate an international emergency response, known as the humanitarian cluster response system, and stand in for the country's beleaguered public health system. Civil servants in the Ministry of Health were agitating for the declaration of a 'national disaster', as they felt that the health system was completely overwhelmed by the epidemic.

By the end of November 2008, three of the country's four major hospitals had shut down, as had the medical school at the University of Zimbabwe. Furthermore, the fourth major hospital was limited to two wards and had no working surgical theatres (Hungwe 2008). As Stanley Midzi explained to me when I asked about the delay between the detection of the outbreak and the instigation of a full-scale humanitarian response,

> I think your question is good because the delay between this rapid escalation of cases between August and September/October. We, as a Department of Epidemiology and Disease Control, were mandated to contain cholera. Within a month, by the end of September, we were clearly seeing that we were getting overwhelmed to a point where we knew with our resources and capacity that we were not able to manage. Me, as a Director of Epidemiology had made a recommendation to the Permanent Secretary so that he could recommend to the Minister of Health that: 'Look, I think it's high time that he considers recommending to the President that he declares a national disaster.'[35]

each geographical or temporal unit and then compared using standard statistical methods.

[35] Stanley Midzi 2015 int.

The refusal to acknowledge the outbreak as a disaster – a highly contentious political choice and the subject of the next chapter – had devastating consequences.

By 2 December, the WHO announced that since August, the Zimbabwean Ministry of Health and Child Welfare had recorded a staggering 11,735 cases of cholera and 484 deaths throughout the country. In some rural areas, cholera mortality rates reached an astonishing 20 to 30 per cent. Additionally, the health crisis contributed to the already large-scale population movement out of Zimbabwe into South Africa (Bolt 2015; Médecins Sans Frontières 2009a). By January 2009, before the peak of outbreak, an estimated 38,000 Zimbabweans had fled into South Africa as a result of cholera, with some migration to other neighbouring countries as well (Edelstein, Heymann, and Koser 2014). The disease made clear how Zimbabwe's crisis had become a burden to the entire region of southern Africa.

Having initially denied the presence of an outbreak, the Zimbabwean government belatedly declared a national emergency in mid-December and finally appealed to the international community for further assistance. The United Kingdom, United States, European Commission, UN agencies, the International Federation of the Red Cross, Oxfam and MSF, among several others, provided funds and technical support. By February 2009, the WHO counted nearly 80,000 suspected cases of cholera and 3,713 deaths as well as 8,000 weekly cases in that month – the peak of the epidemic. At this point, there were 365 cholera treatment centres and units throughout the country. But even with this assistance and attention, WHO officials remained pessimistic about the chances of a quick resolution: 'Given the outbreak's dynamic, in the context of a dilapidated water and sanitation infrastructure and a weak health system, the practical implementation of control measures remains a challenge' (World Health Organization 2009).

The majority (61 per cent) of those who died of cholera failed to reach a cholera treatment facility owing to such factors as 'limited geographical access, lack of commodities such as sugar and salt to make [oral rehydration therapy] at home, soap for hand washing, lack of awareness and access to adequate information and lack of knowledge about how cholera spreads' (World Health Organization/Government of Zimbabwe: Ministry of Health 2011). Additionally, there was no systematic collection of demographic data at the treatment centres, as Ben Henson, a water, sanitation and hygiene specialist from UNICEF who worked in Zimbabwe during the outbreak, explained:

> One of our frustrations from the beginning was that there was very little disaggregation of the data collected out of the treatment centres in terms of age and gender. We requested this time and time again, it just wasn't forthcoming. I'm not saying it was withheld, it just wasn't there. And this was the same coming from the WHO.[36]

'Anecdotally', Henson continued, 'there was an interesting demographic in that a significant number of young men, 18 to 30, were affected.' An internal report from US Centers for Disease Control (CDC) on the outbreak suggested that young men were disproportionately affected because they tended to avoid treatment for the disease and they stayed clear of health promotion campaigns in local communities. Henson interpreted the findings in the following way:

> I don't know what the final document was that [the CDC] eventually produced, I only saw the presentation that they made at the end of their research. Our [UNICEF's] interpretation of that trend without firm evidence was that – and it's one of the reasons that in the current urban programming that UNICEF is supporting through other organisations there's a strong focus on men – men don't want to participate in clubs, men don't go to health clubs, men don't go to hygiene promotion sessions, men are not as clean as children and women or at least women make sure that children are. And this is our interpretation.[37]

By March 2009, the situation started to improve as both the incidence of cases and the case fatality rate began to decline. By late May 2009, WHO had recorded a cumulative total of 98,424 cases of cholera and 4,276 deaths in fifty-five of sixty-two districts since the start of the outbreak,[38] which had had largely abated by mid-2009.

Conclusion

Through a granular analysis of how the cholera outbreak unfolded, this chapter has reinforced Charles Rosenberg's notion of 'configuration' as

[36] Interview, Ben Henson, Harare, 12 November 2015. [37] Ibid.
[38] See Luque Fernández et al. (2011; 2012) for a detailed spatial analysis of the spread of cholera in 2008–09.

a conceptual approach to explaining epidemics. I argued that the cholera outbreak was precipitated and perpetuated by a toxic synergy of the collapse of Zimbabwe's public health delivery system, the failure of the water reticulation systems and a multifaceted urban crisis that included widespread food insecurity and malnutrition. In so doing, I echo Tony Barnett and Alan Whiteside's (2002: 15) aphorism that 'The conditions that facilitate rapid spread of an infectious disease are also, by and large, those that make it hard for societies to respond – and ensure that the impact will be severe.' Crucially, the very existence of the antecedent factors that lead to an outbreak are seldom 'natural'. Thus, as with other major epidemics, the cholera outbreak was a path-dependent process, rooted in real historical decisions and non-decisions, in socio-economic inequality and in political conflicts.

In this chapter, I have used the cholera outbreak not only to demonstrate the multi-level failure of a range of public services but also as an avenue into debates about state institutions in Zimbabwe. The point that the post-2000 transformation in Zimbabwe had catastrophic effects, as illustrated through the outbreak, has now been well made. The state is not a homogenous entity: failures in different public services mutually reinforced each other and reverberated in multiple and sequential ways, thereby showing the ramifications of political choices in the failure of public service delivery.

Cholera created a charged and high-stakes series of political debates about the state, about the legitimacy of the ruling party, about the lives of the people it infected and about the responses of different institutions to it. By giving a thoroughgoing and detailed account of how the cholera outbreak occurred, this chapter has now set the scene for an exploration of the different interpretations and narratives that the epidemic provoked.

3 Emergency Politics

Cholera as a National Disaster

Only when the presence of an epidemic becomes unavoidable is there public admission of its existence. Bodies must accumulate and the sick must suffer in increasing numbers before officials acknowledge what can no longer be ignored. The pattern has repeated itself in century after century.

—Charles Rosenberg, *Explaining Epidemics and Other Studies in the History of Medicine*, 1992

Disease is deliberately caused by the white man to decimate the race, to undermine our well-being, to impoverish and compel us to serve as his labourers. Disease never comes of itself. It is caused.

—Herbert Isaac Ernest Dhlomo, *Malaria*, 1985

The dramatic scale and devastating impact of the cholera epidemic precipitated a political outcry that echoed loudly across a spectrum of institutions. The disease reinforced an image of Zimbabwe as a 'pathological', 'pariah' and 'failed' state, as portrayed by the country's opposition political parties,[1] a host of foreign governments, multiple agencies in the mainstream international media, key organisations in the humanitarian sector and several influential global security and development think tanks (see Taylor 2013). For instance, the Council on Foreign Relations (Patrick 2011: 229) asserted that Zimbabwe's health crisis, epitomised by the cholera epidemic, could be 'attributed to the decay of state institutions and infrastructure' under the 'brutal regime' of the 'despot Robert Mugabe'. Similarly, *The New York Times* blamed Mugabe's government for the cholera crisis because of its avaricious pursuit of 'power and money' (Dugger 2008). Prominent reports by the International Crisis Group (ICG) (2008) and Physicians

[1] Multiple interviews with politicians in the Movement for Democratic Change and other smaller political parties.

for Human Rights (PHR) (Sollom et al. 2009) characterised the Zimbabwean situation, and specifically the cholera outbreak, in terms of 'state failure' and thus as a potential target for military intervention motivated by the 'Responsibility to Protect' (R2P) doctrine. Richard Bourne (2011), a former journalist and a senior research fellow at the Commonwealth Institute at the University of London, wrote a popular account of Zimbabwe's crisis, entitled *Collapse: What Went Wrong in Zimbabwe?* Bourne captured much of this narration about the country succinctly when he wrote: 'No one in 1980 could have predicted that Zimbabwe would become a failed state on such a monumental and tragic scale.'

While the ZANU(PF) government was receiving widespread international condemnation for the multifaceted crisis in the country and President Robert Mugabe was vilified, the regime obstinately refused to acknowledge the overwhelming extent and devastation of cholera for the first three months of the outbreak. Inevitably, however, such political quiescence in the face of accumulating cadavers and the macabre sight of the suffering sick was impossible to maintain. On 4 December 2008, under considerable political and bureaucratic pressure, the Minister of Health at the time, Dr David Parirenyatwa, proclaimed that the cholera epidemic was a national disaster and pleaded for international relief and medical humanitarian assistance. What appeared to be a positive development in the cholera saga was upended only a week later. On 11 December, in a televised address to the nation from Heroes' Acre, President Mugabe shocked many involved in the cholera response when he stated, 'I am happy we are being assisted by others and we have arrested cholera' (cited in Dzirutwe 2008). Turning his attention to the suggestion of military intervention in the country on humanitarian grounds, he added: 'So now that there is no cholera, there is no cause for war anymore' (cited in Dzirutwe 2008).

The controversy did not stop there. The following day, 12 December, the former and now deceased Minister of Information, Dr Sikhanyiso Ndlovu, seized upon the outbreak to launch a 'daring vitriolic attack on the West and accused it of being the source of the cholera' (Musemwa 2010: 195). In charges harking back to the liberation struggle during which the Rhodesian army used biological warfare by spreading anthrax pathogens in weaponised form among guerrilla fighters and rural civilians (Martinez 2002), Ndlovu accused the West of deploying similar tactics in 2008 (BBC 2008). Ndlovu claimed that British secret agents had clandestinely entered the country to spread cholera and anthrax as a biological weapon to bring about regime change in the country.

In this chapter, I examine the manifold ways in which cholera became a terrain of polarised political contestations internationally and nationally. As the foregoing paragraphs indicate, this polarisation reached extreme levels in which blame for the cholera outbreak was cast as a Manichaean opposition, effectively pitting international accusations of 'state failure' against nationalist claims to 'state sovereignty' and even to international conspiracy. I show that through the allocation of culpability for the cholera outbreak, we see a panoply of actors in the ruling party, in opposition parties, in civil society and in the so-called international community making wide-ranging and competing claims about the cholera outbreak and its wider political implications. I suggest that these political contestations arise from the multiple ontologies of the cholera outbreak. I argue that different actors and institutions encountered different forms of the outbreak, and thus they made competing claims about why cholera was an emergency, and they insisted on different, often incompatible modes of action to quell it. The multiple ontologies framework allows us to unpack the category of emergency and apprehend its attendant politics. It allows us to see how cholera presented numerous threats at the same time. It helps us to explain how different actors attempted to command the narrative about the cholera outbreak, to shape public perceptions about its causes and consequences, and to direct collective action in response to it according to their institutional ambitions, political ideologies or world views.

I begin by discussing my use of the titular term for this chapter, 'emergency politics'. Following Jennifer Rubenstein (2015), I define 'emergency politics' as the processes by which many different actors make, contest, accept, ignore and reject a wide array of claims about the interplay of values, threats and human agency in a situation where harm or destruction is at stake. I then illustrate the multiplicity of the cholera outbreak by examining how numerous emergency claims about the disease were made in three major and overlapping areas that I separate out for analytical clarity: humanitarianism, security and governance. Finally, I argue that the political contestations around cholera were deleterious in the extreme. These disagreements undermined engagement between the Zimbabwean and Western governments (Alao 2012) and narrowed down the avenues for third-party diplomatic mediation (Tendi 2014). Moreover, as I elaborate more fully in Chapter 4, the emergency politics of cholera both delayed and then complicated the humanitarian relief effort (Fournier and Whittall 2009).

Commanding the Narrative

At the height of Zimbabwe's hyperinflation and infrastructural collapse, and in the wake of its unprecedented electoral violence, the stand-off between the government and its opposition had huge costs. On 15 September 2008, the Global Political Agreement (GPA), a power-sharing agreement, intended to break the political deadlock created by the contentious presidential election in preceding months, was signed. It was agreed that Robert Mugabe would continue to hold his position as president, despite the violent tactics he adopted to 'win' the 2008 elections. At the same time, the main opposition leader, Morgan Tsvangirai, was appointed Prime Minister. Control of ministries was split across the three main political parties – ZANU(PF), MDC-Tsvangirai (MDC-T) and the smaller MDC-Mutambara (MDC-M) – and constitutional reforms were set out (Hoekman 2013). Nevertheless, the only major point of inter-party agreement was that the disputed elections and economic crisis demanded urgent resolution (Dorman 2016). The precise terms of the settlement that would culminate in a Government of National Unity (GNU) in February 2009, however, were heatedly battled over in a drawn-out, high-level, closed-door process (Dorman 2016; Hoekman 2013).

While the negotiations were under way for the formation of a GNU, the cholera epidemic proceeded apace, progressively revealing itself through astonishing mortality rates and triggering a sense of collective crisis manifest as panic, anger, suspicion and denial as evidenced by newspaper accounts and rumours spreading through the city.[2] For its part, the government remained taciturn about the disease in the early stages of the outbreak. The collapse of the healthcare system severely compromised epidemic monitoring and surveillance, as discussed in the previous chapter, while the political costs of acknowledging the

[2] Interviews with journalists (e.g. Kumbirai Samuriwo), healthcare workers (e.g. Tungamirai Mhuka) and activists (e.g. Hardlife Mudzingwa).

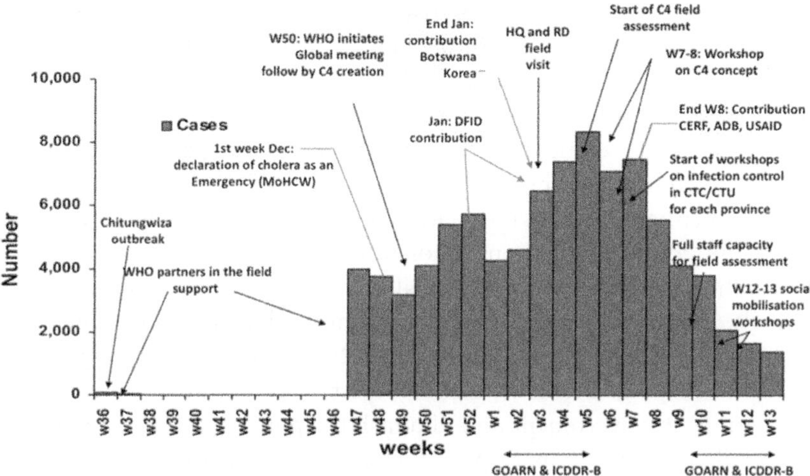

Figure 3.1 Links between cholera response and epidemiological trends.
Source: Joint Cholera Initiative for Southern Africa. On the horizonal axis denoting 'weeks', w36–w52 refer to the last seventeen weeks on 2008, that is, from August to December, while w1–w13 refers to the first thirteen weeks of 2009, that is, from January to March. GOARN is the Global Outbreak Alert and Response Network and ICDDR-B is the International Centre for Diarrhoeal Disease Research, Bangladesh

outbreak were high for the ruling party. A vexatious picture emerged in which a horrific and deadly epidemic was killing people in their hundreds and thousands yet appeared non-existent in official political communication. This is illustrated below in Figure 3.1, which depicts the linkages between cholera's epidemiological trends and the public health response to it. The graph, provided to me by the Ministry of Health, shows a glaring omission of data in the first three months of the outbreak before the disease was declared a disaster.

Why was cholera such a sensitive political issue? How are we to make sense of the political ramifications of acknowledging the disease as a lethal epidemic? The early stages of the outbreak, as rumours and initial reports circulated about its spread, saw a frantic rush among diverse agencies to shape perceptions of and response to cholera through different public narratives. Raising public questions about cholera – where it came from, whom it affected and why it affected them – formed a crucial part of the actions and events that constituted the politics of the epidemic. Different constituencies offered highly contrastive answers to pressing questions like: Where did cholera come from? Who and what was at risk? What could be done to stop it? Finally, who was to blame for the high incidence of infection and death in the townships and beyond?

Opposition politicians insisted that their counterparts in the ruling party were too afraid to acknowledge the disease publicly because, they argued, it would be an admission that ZANU(PF) had 'failed' as a government and needed international assistance to manage the crisis.[3] In the popular imagination,[4] cholera became a tragically apt political metaphor: a symbol of how ZANU(PF) had taken the country backwards, marking a radical departure from its claims to delivering modernising development (see Dorman 2016). For the ruling party, however, laying the blame on 'the West' was a strategy to exculpate its actions in government and diminish the potency of the claim that it had failed to honour its responsibilities of public provision of services, especially those services with existential implications such as water, sanitation and healthcare. In the context of unprecedented electoral violence, economic meltdown and fraught political negotiations to form a coalition government, the cholera outbreak was, in the words of a Harare-based activist, 'one crisis too many'.[5] The stakes around taking responsibility for cholera were clearly very high.

Brian Patrick, a veteran humanitarian aid worker with over thirty years' experience, spoke to me about the implications of any government admitting to having a cholera outbreak within its borders:

> Cholera is one of those words, which causes things to happen when you say it. The two other words – and these are more serious words – that have that effect are famine and genocide. Cholera is the little brother of those big words that change things when you say them. It's because it's such an awful disease, because it spreads so rapidly, because people die in such an appalling way . . . There are all kinds of reasons why the government might not want to announce that there is cholera, and it's very common for countries around the world not to announce that they have cholera . . . cholera makes you look like a badly run, dirty, tin-pot country and that's why people are so afraid of

[3] Multiple interviews with civil servants and opposition politicians e.g. Henry Madzorera, Margaret Dongo and Tendai Biti.

[4] Interviews with residents of Harare's high-density townships, discussed fully in Chapter 6.

[5] Interview, Activist, Harare, 6 October 2015.

it. It damages your reputation, it damages your economy, it damages tourism; it's really bad news to have cholera in your country.[6]

For humanitarian actors, Patrick effectively argues that the declaration of a cholera outbreak constitutes a 'performative speech act' (Buzan, Wæver and Wilde 1999). Its invocation 'does something' – more specifically it grants international humanitarian organisations, both non-governmental and multilateral, legitimacy to intervene in a country on the basis of providing necessary, life-saving emergency relief. Humanitarians act on cholera as a specific type of emergency. However, as Jennifer Rubenstein (2015) writes, an emergency claim can be made by a diverse body of different kinds of actors. An emergency claim, in her view, is simply a claim that a given situation is an emergency. It is made by particular actors against a set of background conditions to given audiences, who then accept, ignore or reject that claim. In turn, emergency politics consists of many different actors making and not making, accepting and rejecting, a wide range of competing and overlapping emergency claims.

> Emergency claimants use speech, writing, visual images, and other strategies to persuade their audience(s) that (i) some person(s), thing(s), or state(s) of affairs are valuable, but (ii) they are threatened with imminent harm or destruction, yet (iii) human agency is capable of preventing or reversing at least some of that harm or destruction. That is, emergency claims are claims about value, threat, and human agency (among other things). (Rubenstein 2015: 102)

In the abstract, if an emergency claim is made successfully, then it shapes the receiving audience's understanding of a given situation, it directs resources or attention to the needs or cause identified by the claimant, it confers new powers or legitimacy to the claimant, or it achieves some combination of all these effects. In reality, of course, not all emergency claims are equal, nor do they exist in isolation: they are conditioned by the power dynamics, social structures and historical context of where, when, how and why they are made.

In the remainder of the chapter, I use Rubenstein's notion of emergency politics as a heuristic tool to examine the multiple ontologies of cholera through a series of contested emergency claims made in relation to humanitarianism, security and governance. By examining

[6] Interview, Brian Patrick, London, 6 July 2015.

emergency claim-making in the cholera outbreak, this chapter gives an analysis of how different actors attempted to command the narrative about cholera, to win over different audiences and to shape how the disease was dealt with based on their experience of the outbreak, on their social and political positions, on their organisational priorities and on their individual and corporate ideologies. These emergency claims ran into conflict with each other repeatedly thereby stalling a response to the outbreak.

In the Name of Humanity

Operating in the context of Zimbabwe's struggling health care system, Médecins Sans Frontières (MSF) was instrumental in addressing the cholera outbreak between August, its official onset, and February, when a fully integrated multi-sectoral response effort was under way. During this period, the organisation reports that its medical teams treated nearly 45,000 patients directly while supporting the treatment of several thousands more through the provision of supplies, logistical support, technical advice and training to Ministry of Health staff (Médecins Sans Frontières 2009a). In the ethos of *témoignage* – MSF's notion of 'witnessing' out of a concern for human suffering (Redfield 2011) – the organisation raised the alarm about the unfolding humanitarian crisis in the country. They issued press statements and emergency reports stating that Zimbabwe's 'political crisis and resultant economic collapse is manifesting in cholera, population movement, hyperinflation, food insecurity, violence and a lack of access to HIV/AIDS treatment and health care more generally' (Médecins Sans Frontières 2009a: 4). MSF bemoaned the government's 'rigid control over aid organisations' (Médecins Sans Frontières 2009b: 4), which hampered the organisation's capacity to deliver emergency medical assessments and interventions. To curb any further avoidable loss of life, MSF advocated the preservation of a 'humanitarian space' in which it could fulfil its duty to rescue:

> Now more than ever, an adequate humanitarian response in Zimbabwe will require an increase in 'humanitarian space' for independent aid organisations to carry out our work. The Zimbabwean government must facilitate independent assessments of need, guarantee that aid agencies can work wherever needs are identified and ease bureaucratic restrictions so that

programmes can be staffed properly and drugs procured quickly. Donor governments and United Nations agencies must ensure that the provision of humanitarian aid remains distinct from political processes. Their policies towards Zimbabwe must not come at the expense of the humanitarian imperative to ensure that malnourished children, victims of violence, and people with HIV/AIDS and other illnesses have unhindered access to the assistance they need to survive. (Médecins Sans Frontières 2009c: 4)

Under the guise of neutrality, MSF spoke of Zimbabwe's 'political crisis' while carefully avoiding the specific mention of actors or institutions responsible for it. Instead, the organisation fought for and jealously guarded its autonomy to deliver emergency relief to those in need.

Around the same time, the Zimbabwe Lawyers of Human Rights (ZLHR), a not-for-profit human rights organisation, took a strikingly different approach in its advocacy for human rights during the cholera outbreak. On 25 September 2008, just over a month after the first official case of cholera had been registered, ZLHR delivered a public statement holding the Zimbabwean government responsible for 'avoidable cholera deaths'.

Zimbabwe Lawyers for Human Rights (ZLHR) is saddened to learn of the unnecessary deaths of sixteen (16) people who have recently succumbed to the devastating effects of cholera. According to two reports published by the state-controlled Herald newspaper this week and confirmed by Health and Child Welfare Minister David Parirenyatwa, 16 people have so far fallen victim to the cholera outbreak in Chitungwiza while 88 people have to date been hospitalized both in the dormitory town and in the capital Harare in just less than a month. The ongoing deaths, *which are a result of official and criminal negligence*, have brought despair to the affected families and communities and the nation at large. It is alarming and quite unusual for such a preventable disease to continue to claim such valuable lives in this day and age. If more than a dozen people have died from cholera in just less than a month, we can only imagine how many more are currently affected by, or at risk of contracting, this avoidable disease. (Zimbabwe Lawyers for Human Rights 2008, emphasis added)

ZLHR's statements were extensively covered in the national news, and the organisation soon became one of the most vocal critics, on the domestic scene, of the government's role in the cholera outbreak. Invoking Article 25 of the Universal Declaration of Human Rights, Article 12 of the International Covenant on Economic, Social and

Cultural Rights, and the African Charter on Human and Peoples' Rights, ZLHR asserted that the government, and through it the local authorities and the Zimbabwe National Water Authority (ZINWA), were accountable for the deaths of the cholera victims because they had collectively failed to provide basic health services, to ensure access to clean running water and sanitation facilities, and to respond swiftly to the disease outbreak.[7] In contrast to MSF's 'neutrality', ZLHR explicitly denounced the government for its 'criminal' action and called for punishment of the actors whom they deemed responsible, as Kumbirai Mafunda from the organisation explained to me:

> I think the government does have an obligation to protect its citizens. There had been early warning signs on this issue. The red buttons were already being pressed prior to the outbreak of this cholera. The government did not even act to put in measures to prevent the outbreak of such a medieval disease in this period that we're living in. That's where you can locate the element of neglect within the government. Had government really acted on the warning signs that were presented, it should have put in structures and preventive measures to contain this disease. But what did we see in 2008? We actually had a Minister of Information – Sikhanyiso Ndlovu, may his soul rest in peace – saying this disease is as a result of the British and the Western governments using biological warfare. What was needed at that time was to put measures in place but the government was in a denial mode prior to the outbreak of cholera. That's where we can start to locate the negligence part on the side of the government. We look at the response part and the priority in terms of allocating resources to deal with the outbreak. What resources were put in place by government? The government was more focused on retaining political power, especially the ZANU(PF), instead of mobilising resources for containing this disease.[8]

Physicians for Human Rights (PHR), an international advocacy group founded on the belief that 'physicians, scientists, and other health professionals possess unique skills that lend significant credibility to the investigation and documentation of human rights abuses' (Physicians for Human Rights 2011), sent a team of four field investigators – Richard Sollom, David Sanders, Chris Beyrer and A. Frank Donaghue – into Zimbabwe in December 2008 to document health-related human rights failures. Working in conjunction with their local chapter, the Zimbabwe

[7] Interview, Kumbirai Mafunda (press officer for ZLHR), Harare, 1 October 2015.
[8] Ibid.

Association of Doctors for Human Rights (ZADHR), the team spent about a week traveling around the country visiting cholera treatment centres and other health facilities. They met with staff in different facets of the health system and spoke extensively with opposition politicians and civil society actors. Despite efforts to remain covert, rumours of the PHR investigation reached official ears. David Sanders described to me how Rick Sollom was confronted by journalists from the Zimbabwe Broadcasting Corporation (ZBC) when he was about to leave the country at the end of the field trip:

> As they pulled [into Harare International Airport], two [Zimbabwe Broadcasting Corporation] TV cameramen immediately descended on [Rick Sollom], started to film him and ask him questions saying, 'We understand that you came here to investigate the cholera epidemic. What have you found?' He did not know how they knew that he was there. We had tried to keep it pretty quiet. While he was standing in line waiting to check in, they continued to interrogate him and he wisely didn't say anything. ... he told us an airport worker sitting behind a desk somewhere just said to him very surreptitiously, 'Sir, I would advise you not to go through immigration. The security branch is waiting there to arrest you on the other side.' So, he came back to where Frank and I were and told us the story. ... We packed up quickly and we headed straight for ... a safe house. We started to pack our stuff and to arrange to leave Zimbabwe by road. We had no intention of going back to the airport. ... We decided not to go out through Beitbridge because we thought that they might pick us up there. We went through the border at Kariba, which is a minor border. ... we got through the border, got to Zambia and had a good few drinks that night. And then, we booked flights back via [Johannesburg].[9]

The story illustrates the sensitivity around reporting about cholera at the time and the government's determination to keep news of cholera contained and retain command of the narrative. Douglas Gwatidzo, a medical doctor and former chair of the Zimbabwe Association of Doctors for Human Rights, corroborated the airport incident,

> I think it was all because of the fears of a potential British or American infiltration. As far as government was concerned, this was an attempt to bring in the foreigners under the guise of wanting to know more about cholera. And as I said, this was after a very contentious, disputed election. The atmosphere was just tense. Any foreign person who would be going

[9] Interview, David Sanders, Johannesburg, 12 September 2015.

around the country gathering information, genuine information on things that were going on would be considered an enemy of the state until proven otherwise. So it's not surprising.[10]

The PHR report, *Health in Ruins: A Man-Made Disaster in Zimbabwe*, was published in January 2009. Pitched as a human rights emergency report with a preface written by Richard J. Goldstone (Former UN Chief Prosecutor, International Criminal Tribunals for the former Yugoslavia and Rwanda), Mary Robinson (Former UN High Commissioner for Human Rights) and Desmond Tutu (Anglican Archbishop Emeritus of Cape Town), the document is a comprehensive and scathing indictment of the Zimbabwean government. PHR accuse Dr Parirenyatwa of instructing the media to turn a blind eye to the number of people who had died or become infected with cholera; they assert that the government intentionally suppressed information regarding increasing malnutrition; and, more broadly, they argue that 'the Mugabe regime has used any means at its disposal, including politicizing the health sector, to maintain its hold on power' (Sollom et al. 2009: iii). Ultimately, the report concludes:

> There is no doubt that egregious, widespread, and systematic violations of human rights have occurred under the Mugabe-led ZANU-PF regime and that death and serious injury to the physical and mental health of Zimbabweans continue unabated. To date, international criminal prosecution has not addressed crimes against humanity in the context of wilful and state-sponsored actions that lead to massive loss of life resulting from, for example, failures to respond to epidemics, active obstruction of humanitarian aid, or the deliberate destruction of health systems. ... The U.N. Security Council, acting pursuant to its authority under Article 41 of the Charter, should enact a resolution referring the crisis in Zimbabwe to the International Criminal Court for investigation and to begin the process of compiling documentary and other evidence that would support the charge of crimes against humanity. (Sollom et al. 2009: 44–45)

In similar fashion, the International Crisis Group (2008) published a report, *Ending Zimbabwe's Nightmare: A Possible Way Forward*, arguing that the Zimbabwe situation had deteriorated to such an extent that its catalogue of human rights abuses and consequent humanitarian crisis, especially the cholera outbreak, posed 'a threat

[10] Interview, Douglas Gwatidzo, Harare, 26 October 2015.

to international peace and security' and 'could itself be characterised as involving the commission of a crime against humanity' (International Crisis Group 2008: 10, 9). As such, ICG charged that Zimbabwe ought to be dealt with according to the 'responsibility to protect' (R2P) norm and that 'coercive military intervention' should be considered to depose Robert Mugabe and his party from power. The report did concede that it would be difficult to garner political will among Zimbabwe's neighbouring countries for a military intervention and that it would be a challenge to mobilise troops for such a mission given the large unmet requirements for UN-mandated missions in the Congo and Darfur and the lack of interest in supporting a UN mission in Somalia.

The respective positions of MSF, ZLHR, PHR and the ICG, among several other NGOs and advocacy groups, share a common and essential concern with humanity expressed in a language of humanitarianism and human rights. However, the very notion of humanity in which these organisations make their claims about the cholera outbreak is deployed with polyvalence resulting in a multitude of possible meanings and inferences. Furthermore, each of these groups was pitching their claims to different audiences including but not limited to the international donor community, multilateral organisations, other humanitarian groups, local civil society activists, national and international courts and so forth. These groups made overlapping and competing emergency claims based on different assertions about the nature of cholera and the threat it presented, on different evaluations of what was at stake, and on different conceptions of how the situation could have been ameliorated.

In pleading for 'humanitarian space' independent of political processes, MSF brings the temporality of a medical emergency to larger social and political problems. The organisation thus does not act with longer-term political consequences in mind, choosing instead to act in the name of immediate, urgent and temporary care and in the name of political neutrality. As Miriam Ticktin (2011) has documented, proponents of this approach to humanitarianism, the so-called 'new humanitarianism', argue that it is the ability to isolate victims in their present crisis, outside of history and politics, that allows humanitarian organisations to work most effectively and to render borders irrelevant in the name of a higher moral injunction to prevent and relieve the suffering of others. Importantly, Peter Redfield (2011) cautions that MSF's 'humanitarian space' is a 'fragile fiction' – one invoked strategically by the organisation and easily disrupted by the wider political context of its operationalisation.

By contrast, ZLHR's emergency claims about the cholera outbreak located the source of threat in the malign negligence of the ZANU(PF) government. For them cholera was a symptom of corruption and malfeasance. They insisted that what was really at stake was more than the lives of people but rather the integrity of a normative conception of the social contract in which the state responsibly delivers public goods to its citizens; and they sought to rectify this situation through the instruments of criminal justice. ZLHR's paradigm of criminal justice identifies blameworthy actors and institutions culpable for the mass suffering of the cholera outbreak and attempts to use local institutions, such as the courts, to hold them accountable to the people of Zimbabwe.

PHR and ICG draw on both medical humanitarianism and international legal paradigms to inform their emergency claims. They construct a 'health–security' nexus in which outbreaks are a threat because they are societally destabilising events capable of compromising the security of nation states. Their vision of how human agency can configure the outcome therefore includes a salient new dimension: the security sector. By invoking the R2P norm, these organisations consider the possibility of military coercion as an immediate remedy to the emergency after which, they argue, an unencumbered medical response could be mobilised to address the needs of cholera's victims while the International Criminal Court – presented as an objective, apolitical arbiter of justice – can mete out punishment to the politicians who presided over the crisis in the first place. Crucially, PHR and ICG called on the 'international community' to be key agents of change, thereby subordinating Zimbabwe's sovereignty to the prerogatives of global governance institutions and norms.

The emergency claims made in the name of humanity during the cholera outbreak, as described above, are born out of its different ontologies. Each of the emergency claims entails a different evaluation of the nature of the threat depending on how each agency encountered cholera and depending on each agency's ideological outlook, politics and mandate. MSF located threat in the disease as a clinical entity, ZLHR identified threat in a lack of accountability from the ruling party resulting in an eminently preventable outbreak, while PHR and

ICG delineated a causal connection between cholera and the evil political machinations of Robert Mugabe. Similarly, the agencies made different assertions of what was at stake: the lives of vulnerable Zimbabweans; the institutions of public order and democracy; the security of the region of southern Africa. And, finally, these agencies advocated entirely different modes of acting on the cholera crisis, through emergency medical relief in the case of MSF, through criminal prosecution of key politicians and state actors in the case of ZLHR, and through international military and judicial intervention and courts in the case of PHR and ICG. These narratives provoked a belligerent counter-narrative in Zimbabwe as I detail in the following section.

Under Siege

An integral part of the Zimbabwe's post-2000 political transformation and re-structuring of the state was a new national narrative espoused by the Zimbabwean government (Hammar, Raftopoulos and Jensen 2003; Ranger 2004; Tendi 2010). This narrative draws motifs from several places including, as Ndlovu-Gatsheni (2009a) describes it, Marxism, Négritude, Pan-Africanism, African neo-traditionalism, and other 'isms'. Disseminated through various media, such as newspapers, political speeches and music, this nationalist discourse – termed 'patriotic history' by Terence Ranger (2004) – retold the story of Zimbabwe's liberation struggle for independence. In this script, the nationalist struggle was 'about fighting men and land ... it was no longer about democracy and rights. Democracy and civil rights were increasingly tarred with that brush of neo-colonialism, cast as un-African and inauthentic, and ceded to the MDC' (Alexander 2010: 193).

In the post-colonial era, so the argument goes, international financial institutions, Western governments and foreign NGOs colluded with the MDC to agitate for political rights and electoral rules, but in reality they collectively aimed to deprive Zimbabweans of their economic rights and their material heritage – that is, the land (Ranger 2004; Alexander 2006, 2010; Tendi 2010). Necessarily, therefore, revolutionary fervour built up, leading to 'spontaneous' land seizures, the Third *Chimurenga*, that began in 2000 and continued until 2003. Britain, the former colonial master worried for her 'kith and kin' in

Zimbabwe, responded by instituting sanctions and trying to 'recolonise' the country. Ultimately, the narrative concludes, these foreign whites worked via local whites and 'puppet' blacks in Zimbabwe, like those in the MDC. 'Puppet' blacks, or 'sellouts', had forgotten their history and their land, and were working to sabotage its reclamation.

Patriotic history feeds ZANU(PF)'s long-standing, historically rooted 'siege mentality': the idea that the country is under relentless threat and that the ruling party must use its security apparatus in a range of political, economic and social spheres to act as an ongoing vanguard for Zimbabwe's perpetual liberation struggles (Alao 2012). Eldred Masunungure, professor of political science at the University of Zimbabwe, put it to me thus:

> [T]he interpretation of national security now is so broad that it would be safer to say what is not a national security threat! … The primacy to maintain power is what propelled government to define almost everything as a national security threat. … Most institutions are under surveillance because of the broad interpretation of national security. I'm not sure there is any policy area that is unaffected or not been defined in terms of national security. Everything is interpreted in national security terms. The military intelligence is a very large department. It is a very large branch in the Defence Forces. And it was enlarged post-2000 and some of the best brains here [at the University of Zimbabwe] are recruited to military intelligence and the [Central Intelligence Organisation]. I was chair of the department and they would come and say, 'we want your best ten students to recruit into the national security.' They would do so in other departments. The strengthening of the security apparatuses both in terms of analysis and in terms of resources. It betrays the priorities of the government that lean unambiguously toward national security and the maintenance of peace and order in the country. … It dovetails with the general political psychology of being under a permanent threat, of being in permanent danger from an imperialist invasion with a regime-change agenda.[11]

The health–security nexus drawn by PHR and ICG was inverted by parts of the ZANU(PF) government in ways consistent with the discursive practices of patriotic history and the party's preoccupation with national security. Most notorious in this respect was the statement by former Minister of Information, Sikhanyiso Ndlovu, at a press conference on 12 December:

[11] Interview, Eldred Masunungure, Harare, 30 October 2015.

> Cholera is a calculated racist terrorist attack on Zimbabwe by the unrepentant former colonial power [Britain] which has enlisted support from its American and Western allies so that they can invade the country, install their stooge who will allow them to repossess our resources ... British operatives are in the country now under disguise and have increased cholera and anthrax seeding. There has been a replanting of cholera and anthrax ... This is a serious biological and genocidal warfare on our people by the British, still fighting to recolonize Zimbabwe. (cited in BBC 2008)

We can thus see the health–security nexus being simultaneously invoked as a basis for international humanitarian intervention *and* as a claim to safeguarding national sovereignty. To paraphrase Rahul Rao (2013), what is being contested here is a spatial allocation of culpability in which, on one hand, problems are represented as arising from local dynamics internal to the putatively dysfunctional states that are the objects of humanitarian intervention, while the 'international' is read as a sanitised space populated by heroic actors ready to rescue people in these benighted locales. On the other hand, nationalist voices valorise state sovereignty by exaggerating the risks of neo-colonial predation by external actors and obscuring their culpability of states in impeding the enjoyment of self-determination by their societies. Rao's insight illustrates one of the fundamental ways in which the cholera outbreak was discursively constructed and contested as the disease was mapped onto opposing narratives of Zimbabwean state sovereignty against claims of state failure.

The ZANU(PF) regime launched an aggressive media campaign through the state's mouthpiece, *The Herald* newspaper, to portray the cholera outbreak as an attack on Zimbabwe from 'the West'. Blessing-Miles Tendi (2010) has argued that media strategies of this character were critical to popularising patriotic history in the public domain. He highlights how nationalist public intellectuals, for instance Tafataona Mahoso, have been arguing in national media that Zimbabwe's sovereignty has been threatened by Western imperialism since the Third *Chimurenga* started. According to Mahoso, American foreign policy in the aftermath of the September 11 attacks on the World Trade Centre was driven by 'evil', and the 'US–UK terror war' was a pretext for global imperialism. Mahoso presented the American and British condemnation of Zimbabwe's 2002 presidential election as 'not free and fair' because of a resurgent Western imperialism bent on toppling governments it found unfavourable (Tendi 2010: 25).

West: Substituting guns for drugs in Zim cholera war
'US masterminded cholera outbreak'
AXIS OF EVIL . . .
Cholera: West's latest weapon on Zimbabwe

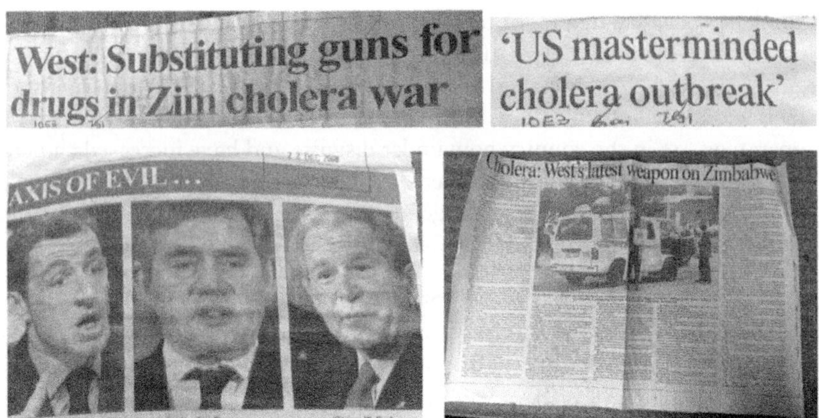

Figure 3.2 Headlines in *The Herald* about cholera in December 2008.
Source: The Herald archives in Harare

Figure 3.2 shows a small selection of cholera-related headlines in *The Herald* to this same effect in December 2008.

A Canada-based blogger and political commentator, Stephen Gowans, published an opinion piece in *The Herald* on 20 December, entitled 'Cholera: West's Latest Weapon on Zimbabwe', which can be seen in Figure 3.2. Gowans (2008) writes that state officials from the West called for Mugabe to step down from power and that 'the crisis is directly linked to Mugabe, its solution to Tsvangirai, but it's never said what Mugabe has done to cause the crisis, or how Tsvangirai's ascension to the presidency will make it go away'. With rhetorical flourish, Gowans makes the case that ZANU(PF)'s military intervention in the Democratic Republic of the Congo in the late 1990s, its rejection of a pro–foreign investment economic restructuring programme from the international financial institutions, and its policies towards land reform were parts of a strategy of revolutionary resistance to 'imperialism' and 'neoliberalism'. For these reasons, the country was punished by a self-interested and venal West through an economically debilitating sanctions programme – to wit the United States' *Zimbabwe Democracy and Recovery Act*. The sanctions, in Gowans's narrative, were both tantamount to an act of war and led directly to the cholera outbreak:

The cholera outbreak [in Zimbabwe] has a parallel in the outbreak of cholera in Iraq following the Gulf War. Thomas Nagy, a business professor

> at George Washington University, cited declassified documents in the September 2001 issue of *The Progressive* magazine showing that the United States had deliberately bombed Iraq's drinking water and sanitation facilities, recognizing that sanctions would prevent Iraq from rebuilding its water infrastructure and that epidemics of otherwise preventable diseases, cholera among them, would ensue. Washington, in other words, deliberately created a humanitarian catastrophe to achieve its goal of regime change. There is a direct parallel with Zimbabwe – the only difference is that the United States uses the Zimbabwe Democracy and Economic Recovery Act – that is, sanctions of mass destruction – in place of bombing. (Gowans 2008)

Much like the nationalist public intellectuals, identified and analysed by Tendi (2010: 35), Gowans also spun a conspiracy theory, used changing international affairs to explain local politics, exploited Western hypocrisy to delegitimise human rights, and eulogised Mugabe as strategies for defending and supporting ZANU(PF). Gowans was exceptionally fluent and coherent with his article, written in the same vein as others written to buttress patriotic history, playing on plausible scenarios and legitimate grievances over Western human rights double standards, which made it persuasive (Tendi 2010: 35).

Journalists working for *The Herald* newspaper in the mid-2000s told me about the strategies used by the Ministry of Information in 2008 to manage the government's suffering reputation in light of the political-economic and humanitarian crises. A former editor at *The Herald*, Kumbirai Samuriwo, described this period of time in the following way: '[W]e were supposed to portray a positive picture of Zimbabwe. We were not supposed to say that there are problems, only challenges.'[12] Instead of probing deeper into stories unfolding around the country, the newspaper's journalists 'had to cover up some of these bad things that were happening in the country'. This strategy fits with what Tendi (2010: 24) calls a 'conspiracy of silence':

> A different type of conspiracy, the conspiracy of silence, was also an integral part of the nationalist public intellectuals' written material. Historical events that blemished ZANU(PF)'s 'unimpeachable' *Chimurenga* time and post-independence record were never articulated in the public sphere. While maintaining a conspiracy of silence on the post-colonial state's immoderations and its various deficiencies, the nationalist public intellectuals engaged in selective historical moralism about the evils of the colonial state.

[12] Interview, Kumbirai Samuriwo, Harare, 16 September 2015.

Moreover, Samuriwo told me that 'there was even victimisation if you tried to do your work in a professional manner'. In mid-2008, he was given a three-month suspension for 'portraying the opposition too much in a positive manner'. Samuriwo explained that he violated the directives from his ministerial superiors – state officials, the permanent secretary and the minister himself – in his coverage of the crisis by not giving the appropriate spin to the stories: 'We were supposed to blame sanctions, Britain, and the opposition. That was the situation during that time.'

Another journalist, Brian Lunga, a former employee of the Zimbabwe Broadcasting Corporation (ZBC) but working as a freelance journalist in 2008, spoke of the difficulties of covering the cholera outbreak because of the government's control of journalists and suppression of information:

> At that time ... anybody who was working as a freelance journalist or was working for foreign media, you were treated with certain stereotypes. They would call you an enemy of the state. Anything negative ... that you reported would make you an enemy of the state. That's the kind of challenge we had. I used to work for ZBC but I left ZBC way back in 2006. When this happened, I had already started working as a freelance journalist and I was working for foreign media. If you want to seek for comments from authorities as a freelance journalist they would not accept you because of what you are trying to probe, what you are trying to get information about is sensitive to them and they would think you want to go and convey negative information about the country. ... Even getting into the centres, it was some sort of guerrilla tactics for you to get an overall picture of what was happening, the people who are suffering. ... In early 2009 ... Tsvangirai was one person who would go into the centres to see what was happening. At that time, he was so hungry to be in the media so we would take advantage of that. We would go as an entourage and we would be part of his team. That's how we would then get the opportunity to go in.[13]

Without a political entourage, it was very difficult to access the cholera treatment centres. As Lunga describes, 'if you want to go on your own and try and find information, they would not allow you because at those same centres, you would have secret service stationed there, police stationed there, government officials stationed there.' Once confronted by these agents, reporters would be quizzed aggressively:

[13] Interview, Brian Lunga, Harare, 24 September 2015.

'where are you coming from? who are you are reporting for? which station or which newspaper is going to publish this?' This silencing of an independent media, Lunga laments, meant that it was extremely difficult 'to get the information out so that you get humanitarian assistance coming in'.

One of the most revealing attempts to command the narrative around cholera, in terms of the length to which the government went to hide the epidemic from full public view, was a scandal that broke out in the UN offices in Zimbabwe. Georges Tadonki, head of the United Nations Office for the Coordination of Humanitarian Affairs (UNOCHA) in Zimbabwe in 2008, was removed from his post in early 2009 by Agostinho Zacarias, then the UN's country chief (Rosen 2013). Tadonki subsequently brought a wrongful termination claim against the UN after his dismissal. This claim culminated in a UN tribunal in Johannesburg on 26 February 2013, during which it was determined that Tadonki had been wrongfully fired after he attempted to warn headquarters of the cholera outbreak. During the tribunal, it was formally established that Zacarias enjoyed a close relationship with various ZANU(PF) leaders. Zacarias had fought alongside ZANU nationalists when the party was in exile in Mozambique during the liberation struggle. In the course of his UN posting in Zimbabwe, Zacarias 'would spend most of his social time with a Mr. Nicholas Goche, an old ZANU-PF politburo member and former head of the Central Intelligence Organization from 2000 to 2004' (cited in Rosen 2013). This closeness, Tadonki argued, spurred a wilful ignorance of the country's deteriorating conditions. Indeed, the tribunal's judges concluded that Zacarias's closeness to ZANU(PF) made it impossible for Tadonki to carry out his duties as head of UNOCHA. They wrote the following in their report of the tribunal:

> There was a humanitarian drama unfolding and people were dying. Part of the population had been abandoned and subjected to repression. The issue between [Tadonki] and the HC [Zacarias] was to what extent these humanitarian concerns should be exposed and addressed and the risk that there was of infuriating the Mugabe government. Matters started to sour when the Applicant started doing his job. RC/HC Zacarias preferred that the Applicant remain quiet. If he remained quiet, OCHA at headquarters would say he was not doing his job. Therefore while silence would bring him trouble from OCHA, noise would infuriate the RC/HC. When the Applicant started organizing a forum made up of the NGOs, the United Nations and the

donors to discuss the situation in Zimbabwe without the approval of RC/HC Zacarias and to achieve a common understanding of the humanitarian situation, the RC/HC became angry. (cited in Rosen 2013)

When I spoke with Goldberg Mangwadu, Director of Environmental Health in the Ministry of Health and Child Welfare, he insisted that part of the delay in declaring cholera a national disaster was that to do so would mean conceding that the 'West's attack' on Zimbabwe was proving successful. Following the internal logic of patriotic history, Mangwadu complained that, instead of helping Zimbabwe, western governments 'were waiting for Zimbabweans to die! That's what they wanted! And then say look at the government of Zimbabwe, it has failed.' The interview aggravated him severely: with palpable anger, he explained to me that 'the end of severe sanctions is a catastrophic outbreak like what happened in Zimbabwe with cholera. That's exactly what they were looking for and wanted.'[14]

Stanley Midzi, former Director of Disease Control and Epidemiology at the Ministry of Health and Child Welfare, similarly spoke to me about how sanctions had produced misery in Zimbabwe and created a political dilemma about whether to acknowledge the cholera outbreak as a national disaster:

> [T]he country was going through sensitive political problems where the government, which was under serious sanctions, did not want to acknowledge that the sanctions were working and now producing results. Obviously, those countries which had imposed sanctions were actually expecting such effects so that they could influence political changes in their favour. But the government was behaving in a macho way where, clearly, they could see that they were in trouble, but they couldn't acknowledge it. To them, it would be to acknowledge failure, that they have failed to manage.[15]

The UNOCHA scandal and the silencing of journalists as well as the commentaries of Sikhanyiso Ndlovu, Stephen Gowans, Goldberg Mangwadu and Stanley Midzi blend political considerations with strategic and ideological discourses of patriotic history to make very different kinds of emergency claims about cholera as compared to those discussed in the preceding section. Ndlovu went as far as saying

[14] Interview, Goldberg Mangwadu, Harare, 17 September 2015.
[15] Interview, Stanley Midzi, Harare, 22 September 2015.

that cholera was a direct attack on Zimbabwe, that the pathogen was literally used as a weaponised bacteriological agent. He legitimated this position by referring back to the Rhodesian's use of bacteriological and chemical weapons during the liberation struggle (Martinez 2002). The other figures whom I have quoted advanced the view that cholera was part of an indirect attack on Zimbabwe; it was a consequence of severe sanctions that crippled the country's social services. What was at stake were the lives of ordinary people, who had become casualties of the West's unrelenting imperialist campaign against Zimbabwe. And consistent with patriotic history, Zimbabwe's political sovereignty and economic self-determination were also at stake, hence the supposed fear that to admit to cholera would be to admit that the state was unable to manage this outbreak on its own and would have to surrender some of its authority to an international humanitarian apparatus, based largely in the West. Thus, they asserted that cholera crises could have been resolved through apolitical medical intervention, the cessation of sanctions and the ongoing rule of ZANU(PF) – after all, to hand over political rule to the opposition would be illegitimate if it was facilitated, as they claim, by a vicious sanctions regime and a biological attack from outside interests.

The cholera outbreak is another empirical example of a dynamic elucidated by Tendi (2010: 177–80) in which the ZANU(PF) government clashed with its external critics, particularly European governments, about sovereignty and the political transformations in the country since the Third *Chimurenga*.

> Sovereignty is considered an invaluable means of self defence against external intrusion, which is viewed with deep suspicion given Africa's legacy of colonial conquest and exploitation. Colonialism was the last major Western intervention in Africa, and its harmful legacies taint the morality of Western intervention and interference. ... Africa and Europe have different understandings of sovereignty. Grasping the historical reasons for these differences allows us to appreciate that Europe and Africa viewed the Third *Chimurenga* through opposed prisms. The African prism prioritised sovereignty over human rights, while the opposite is true for the European prism. ... By evoking Africans' memory of the colonial experience, the ZANU(PF) government sidestepped addressing its human rights violations.

To understand further the polarisation between the views presented in the humanitarian section vis-à-vis the views outlined in this section, I draw on Tendi's (2014) critique of the discourses between Britain and Zimbabwe during the 'crisis years'. Using the metaphor of 'mutual demonisation', Tendi delineates a distinction between normative and instrumental demonisation. Britain's demonisation of Mugabe and ZANU(PF) was normative – that is, it drew on a set of moral beliefs about its foreign policy to 'do good' in Africa. By contrast, instrumental demonisation underlines the agency of Mugabe and ZANU(PF), who found it useful to demonise Britain, and the West, in order to serve domestic agendas. Demonisation of Britain was useful for Mugabe, particularly insofar as ZANU(PF) portrayed the opposition MDC as a party formed and controlled by the British government and thus an illegitimate voice when critiquing the mismanagement of the cholera outbreak. For Mugabe, the MDC was 'evil' by association with Britain: '[w]e cannot discuss with allies of the West. The devil is the devil and we have no idea of supping with the devil' (cited in Tendi 2014: 1264). Associating the MDC with the 'evil' British government, Tendi concludes, was part of wider endeavours to undermine domestic opposition and seal off Thabo Mbeki's attempts to mediate a meaningful negotiation between the ruling party and the MDC about the formation of a power-sharing government, which the then–South African president viewed as a means of resolving part of the Zimbabwean crisis. Similarly, ZANU (PF) cleverly presented human rights as a Trojan horse by which imperialism represents itself as the establisher of the good society, championing 'oppressed subjects' as objects of protection from their national rulers.

Alao (2012) argues that 'the West', through its demonisation of Mugabe, was feeding the regime's obduracy because, once the stand-off started, Mugabe came under pressure from his party and the army leadership not to capitulate. This began a 'blinking competition' in which the Zimbabwean people were the victims (Alao 2012: 184). This 'blinking competition' added to the polarisation between the ruling party and its political rivals in the negotiation process of the GNU. As a hard-hitting statement from the South African cabinet asserted, Zimbabwe's cholera crisis was exacerbated by the stalled formation of a government of national unity between ZANU(PF) and the MDC parties, indicating that the deadlock and political polarisation were exacerbating the country's humanitarian and economic crisis. Part of the statement read:

Cabinet is extremely concerned about the political impasse that is creating a humanitarian crisis in Zimbabwe. The reported outbreak of cholera in parts of that country is a clear indication that ordinary Zimbabweans are the true victims of their leaders' lack of political will and failure to demonstrate seriousness to resolve the political impasse. The Government is disappointed to note that political interests have taken priority at the expense of the lives of ordinary Zimbabweans. South Africa calls on the leaders of Zimbabwe to take urgent steps to finalise the amendments to their constitution, the allocation of the remaining Cabinet posts and the formation of a representative Government without any further delay and before the situation of ordinary Zimbabweans degenerates any further. No amount of political disagreement can ever justify the suffering that ordinary Zimbabweans are being subjected to at the moment. Like SADC [Southern African Development Community], South Africa would like to see a political settlement sooner rather than later so that the region could start focusing on the most urgent measures needed to rebuild Zimbabwe's economy.[16]

The formulations of the cholera outbreak as humanitarian crisis, as a human rights issue and as a security threat were inverted by nationalists in the Zimbabwean government to present these claims as an illegitimate challenge to the country's sovereignty. However, ZANU (PF)'s presentation of the cholera outbreak did not go unchallenged in domestic politics. This opens a third avenue of analysis: competing claims about legitimacy to govern Zimbabwe between the ruling party and the opposition parties.

'Failed' Governance

As noted at the start of this chapter, the notion that Zimbabwe was a 'failed state' became something of a truism in much Western journalism and policy analysis about Zimbabwe in the 2000s. From this perspective, I have argued that the cholera epidemic was couched in a narrative centred on state collapse caused by venal political leadership intent on holding on to power at all costs. Undoubtedly, phenomena such as hyperinflation and extreme deprivation, a precarious and violent political situation, a precipitous fall in life expectancy rates and the cholera outbreak all provided the ingredients for a gripping story about the failure of yet another African state.

16 South African Information Services, 'Statement on Cabinet Meeting of 19 November 2008'.

As my interviews indicate, the notion of 'failure' – used to capture the ruling party's shortcomings in governance, social service delivery, economic performance and public-sector management – was central to the dynamics of blame and denial during the cholera outbreak on the national political scene. Many of my interlocutors in opposition politics firmly believed that for Robert Mugabe and ZANU(PF) to broadcast the full extent and impact of the cholera outbreak, to acknowledge that the national health system could not cope with the epidemic, and to request international assistance, especially from 'the West', was to admit to having failed as a government. Professor Eldred Masunungure articulated this view well:

> In respect of the cholera outbreak, I think the state was unwilling 1) to accept the gravity of the problem and 2) the political leadership of this country is an arrogant political leadership. It rarely admits that it has failed or it is being regarded as failing. . . . The political leadership did not think the cholera outbreak deserved priority in terms of the allocation of resources to deal with that problem. I think the delay was deliberate. They did not want to attract undue, adverse attention internationally. And, it would be a reflection of failure: that the Zimbabwe state is unable to deliver on the services side therefore both the political leadership and the state have failed. Robert Mugabe, our president, is a proud man, a proud politician. He's arrogant. The last thing he will admit is failure. It's part of the equation that explains what happened between August and December.[17]

For opposition politicians the cholera outbreak was, in the words of Tendai Biti (the former Secretary-General of the MDC and later Minister of Finance in the GNU), 'one of the many fingerprints of real collapse'.[18] Biti added that, 'Diseases like cholera are the product of failure. State failure. They don't happen in modern societies anymore. If ZANU acknowledges cholera, it is an admission of failure on their part.' Along the same lines, Margaret Dongo, co-founder of the National Liberation War Veterans Association and the opposition party the Zimbabwe Union of Democrats, and a former Member of Parliament, told me that it is impossible to grasp the mishandling of the cholera outbreak without appreciating it as a result of poor governance

[17] Eldred Masunungure 2015 int. [18] Tendai Biti 2015 int.

and a crumbling economy: '[A]nd you ask yourself how and why had it crumbled? It's because of the leadership. We're talking about a situation where we have serious corruption, maladministration of the economy, and this mentality of putting power before the people.'[19] Dr Henry Madzorera, an MDC politician and Minister of Health during the GNU, explained the government's unwillingness to declare the cholera outbreak a national disaster as follows:

Well, what we know is that our government is not easily ready to accept that there is a problem, particularly if the problem that they are going to admit to points to a failure of government, a failure to run the economy, a failure to run the politics of the land, a failure to provide basic services. They don't want to admit to anything that points a finger at them as having failed. They want to appear to the people to be macho, to be managing all the time, they don't want to admit to any weaknesses. I would like to suspect that perhaps the Minister of Health [David Parirenyatwa] may have wanted to issue a statement earlier but that he was prevented by the system from doing so because the system had and has its own pride. They won't admit easily to failing. That has been the theme since 1980. We still have the same problem. Right now, we have problems, they will not admit to the problems. But they will say, 'we are managing', 'it's sanctions', 'sanctions are hitting us hard'. But sanctions don't cause cholera. It's failure to provide water and sanitation to the people. I pin it down to that one thing: the pride of the government. We might add their ineptitude in dealing with the crisis. Their concern is politics, not health, not economics. They are more concerned with power, being in control. And if a statement they're going to issue is going to diminish their control, their power, they will not issue that statement even if it is beneficial to the nation.[20]

The view that the government was unwilling to acknowledge the cholera outbreak for fear of admitting to failure, and thereby losing political power, was repeated to me by residents of Harare's high-density township where cholera was most severe. I discuss this more fully in Chapter 5, but the following vignette is indicative. James Munyaradzi, an NGO worker and resident of the dormitory town of Chitungwiza on the outskirts of Harare, told me about a conversation concerning cholera and politics in late 2008 that he had in a local bar

19 Interview, Margaret Dongo, Harare, 6 November 2015.
20 Interview, Henry Madzorera, Kwekwe, 16 October 2015.

with a member of the ZANU(PF) negotiating team involved in the political discussions for a coalition government. He quoted his drinking companion as saying, 'We can't admit that there is cholera because the opposition will use it against us.' Munyaradzi recounted how this conversation made clear to him that 'politics took centre stage at the expense of public health and people died. Nobody wanted to take responsibility. If you admit it, then you're taking responsibility. Nobody wanted to take responsibility.'[21]

For opposition politicians, the government's cover-ups, suppression of information and persecution of whistle-blowers during the cholera outbreak effectively conform to what Stanley Cohen (2001) calls 'implicatory denial' – what is denied or minimised are not the facts, or even their conventional interpretation, but the psychological, moral or political implications that typically follow. Unlike literal denial (repudiation of the facts) or interpretive denial (distorted interpretations of the facts), knowledge itself is not at issue in implicatory denial, but rather doing the 'right' thing with this knowledge. As Cohen (2001: 9) puts it, 'These are matters of mobilisation, commitment and involvement. There is a strong sense, though, in which inaction is associated with denial – whether it comes from not-knowing or knowing but not caring.' Douglas Gwatidzo also suggested in an interview that the government was contending with 'implicatory denial':

> If you were to talk one on one with health workers in government, including those in positions of authority, they would express appreciation of the size of the disaster at hand. But I think the difficult part was how to manage the political implications of whatever position you would have taken. I think deep down the majority of professionals in the Ministry [of Health] and in government knew that we had a crisis on our hands but having to divorce that from the politics of the day, that was the difficulty that they were facing.[22]

The emergency claims from the opposition voices therefore suggest that the true threat was a toxic combination of ZANU(PF)'s incompetence, arrogance, denialism and corruption; what was at stake was the

[21] Interview, James Munyaradzi, Harare, 18 December 2015.
[22] Douglas Gwatidzo 2015 int.

governance of the country and management of the public sector; and the crisis could have been resolved through a change of political leadership.

Ultimately, the outbreak of cholera drew poignant attention to the vulnerability of communities affected by the disease. For the MDC, the horrific deaths caused by cholera, especially of its supporters, pushed the party to speed up the negotiations over the implementation of a Global Political Agreement – brokered by the Southern Africa Development Community (SADC) – with their erstwhile political enemies. As Tendai Biti recalls, the cholera epidemic was part of 'the manifold crisis'; there was 'a crisis in the health sector, there was a crisis in social services. It was clear to us. We had to put Zimbabwe first and find a political solution that will mitigate the suffering of our people across the board.'[23]

Conclusion

In this chapter, I have examined the plurality of ways in which cholera became a site of political contestation nationally and internationally. Using Rubenstein's theory of emergency politics, I looked at how a range of actors made different claims about cholera, based on different evaluations of threat, value and agency in three principal domains: humanitarianism, security and governance. The theory of emergency politics thus helped to illuminate how cholera instantiated a wide matrix of concerns as well as 'a frantic competition to shape public perceptions' (Venugopal and Yasir 2017: 5). By showing how different emergency claims were made about cholera, the multiple ontologies of cholera become apparent. The high-stakes politics of the epidemic lies, to a great extent, in its multiple ontologies. Each of the actors I have discussed attempted to advance their own version of cholera as a basis for action, based on their own experiences, politics, ideologies and agendas. Unsurprisingly, such contested versions of cholera made it extremely difficult to find common ground on which the government, its opposition, civil society and the humanitarian community could meet to address the epidemic. In this way, the multiple ontologies of cholera undermined a shared understanding of the problem and what

[23] Biti 2015 int.

to do about it, and they created a series of stand-offs between the political protagonists in this saga during which time Zimbabweans were 'dying like flies'.[24] The next chapter looks at how a complex assemblage of institutions negotiated this political impasse and implemented a medical humanitarian response to the epidemic.

[24] Interview, Tsitsi, Harare, 17 August 2015.

4 The Salvation Agenda

Medical Humanitarianism and the Response to Cholera

None the less, he knew that the tale he had to tell could not be one of a final victory. It could be only the record of what had had to be done, and what assuredly would have to be done again in the never-ending fight against terror and its relentless onslaughts, despite their personal afflictions, by all who, while unable to be saints but refusing to bow down to pestilences, strive their utmost to be healers.

—Albert Camus, *The Plague*, 1947

Amidst all the recriminations for the cholera outbreak and the deaths left in its wake, a humanitarian response to the disease was slowly forged by an extraordinary assemblage of institutions and actors. The patchwork of agencies involved in the response galvanised around wide-ranging moral and political discourses and imperatives to deliver public health. Zimbabwean civil servants like Dr Portia Manangazira in the Ministry of Health and Madzudzo Pawadyira, the director of the Civil Protection Unit in the Ministry of Local Government, articulated to me their commitment to restoring the reputation and legitimacy of the nation's bureaucracies through a proficient and compassionate technical response. In Dr Manangazira's words, 'Mine is just to say how best do you manage the system. ... For us as the Ministry of Health ... we promote human health ... we continue to promote health when those things are no longer so well [politically].'[1]

The Harare-based Pentecostal mega-church, Celebration Ministries International, publicly declared their allegiance to cholera victims. As part of their Christian commitment to bear witness to the power and love of God, the church launched a major medical outreach programme – founded on an ethos of voluntarism, public service and proselytising – to treat people with cholera and conduct health promotion campaigns for vulnerable communities. The church eschewed

[1] Portia Manangazira 2015 int.

politics emphasising instead the need to save bodies from cholera and souls from damnation. As Tom Deuschle, the American founder and senior pastor of the church, put it to me, 'Our loyalty is not to a particular constituency but to humanity and to the work of God. What we cared about was saving lives and ending suffering. As far as I'm concerned, your politics are minor compared to your eternity.'[2] At the same time, a diverse range of international humanitarian groups and NGOs also intervened in the outbreak, espousing the secular humanitarian values of responding to abject need based on an ostensibly shared, egalitarian humanity and a moral imperative to relieve suffering (see for example: Fassin 2007a; Redfield and Bornstein 2011; Ticktin 2011). As Steven Maphosa, the director of the WHO's Cholera Command and Control Centre during the outbreak, observed, 'the issue was response and saving lives ... What we did notice was that NGOs by their nature, they go right down ... to where the action is ... they did a lot of work in saving lives out there.'[3]

When writing about humanitarianism, it is far too tempting and far too limiting to adopt either a posture of excessive reverence or of relentless critique in characterising how relief workers of various descriptions attend to those struck by a disaster such as the cholera outbreak (see Redfield 2005). A more interesting question is: What political dynamics emerge from such circumstances? Responses to the outbreak came in a variety of forms from disparate actors, motivated by different forms of responsibility and civic commitment, and predicated on multiple, often competing understandings of the nature of the cholera crisis. However, as I argue in this chapter, these heterogeneous positions converged on the ineluctable and morally unimpeachable logic of 'saving lives'. I call this logic 'the salvation agenda'. I borrow the term from Alex de Waal's (2006: 63) inquiry into the global humanitarian approach to AIDS in Africa, where he defines the salvation agenda as 'a belief that a combination of money, technology and goodwill can solve any problem'. To this definition I add that the very notion of salvation as the 'preservation or deliverance from ruin, harm or loss'[4] became the *telos* – that is, the ultimate aim – of the humanitarian response to cholera. Crucially, the salvation agenda's command

[2] Interview, Tom Deuschle, Harare, 15 November 2015.
[3] Stephen Maphosa 2015 int.
[4] Oxford Dictionary of English, 'Salvation'. *Oxford Dictionary of English*. Oxford University Press, 2010.

over the predisposing, precipitating and perpetuating factors that led to the cholera outbreak was ever precarious and unsure.

In this chapter, I illustrate the salvation agenda in the following ways. First, I discuss how such an agenda came to be seen as imperative by detailing eyewitness accounts of the bodily experience of cholera and the pathetic medical care available in Zimbabwe's failing health system. The writing in this section is quite graphic. Disturbing bodily experiences of faecal incontinence and unrestrained vomiting and horrific images of dead bodies piled on top of each other in makeshift mortuaries were foundational to the moral imagination of relief workers, development professionals and bureaucrats who insisted that 'something must be done'[5] to end this suffering. Second, I argue that the life-or-death immediacy of such experiences – compounded by the political impasse discussed in the preceding chapter – attenuated a political and structural response to the outbreak. The urgency of the situation focussed attention on addressing the clinical needs of patients with cholera and removing the most proximal causes of the outbreak. In other words, the necessary, short-term delivery of intravenous fluid hydration in the clinic and the distribution of water purification tablets in the community eclipsed the need to attend to the long-term and multi-scalar political-economic determinants of the cholera crisis. I demonstrate this mode of action by looking at the formation and politics of the WHO Cluster Approach in Zimbabwe, the medical outreach work of Celebration Ministries International and the disaster relief provided by international humanitarian organisations.

I argue that what we see in the salvation agenda is something akin, though not identical, to James Ferguson's (1990) 'anti-politics machine'. For Ferguson, development interventions and discourse entail, among other things, a representation of social and economic life, which denies 'politics'. This development apparatus is an 'anti-politics machine': it depoliticises 'everything it touches, everywhere whisking political realities out of sight, all the while performing, almost unnoticed, its own pre-eminently political operation of expanding bureaucratic state power' (Ferguson 1990: xv). The salvation agenda did not deny the political per se, but rather it knowingly,

[5] Interviews with Pastor Tom Deuschle, medical volunteers such as Dr Andrew Reid and Dr Tungamirai Mhuka, development workers such as Ajay Paul, and bureaucrats such as Steven Maphosa and Stanley Midzi.

often explicitly bypassed the political in favour of the technical and the ethical. However, unlike Ferguson's anti-politics machine, the salvation agenda did not surreptitiously expand bureaucratic state power. Instead the salvation agenda undermined Zimbabwe's bureaucracies by yielding much command of the medical humanitarian cholera response to non-state entities with the justification that something had to be done to stop the emergency and that state bureaucracies were incapacitated and ill-equipped to deliver. As will become clear throughout the chapter, the salvation agenda thus clashed with local pre-existing views and normative expectations of the Zimbabwean state as the primary vehicle for the delivery of development and it clashed with the hopes of more enduring solutions to the country's crisis of which cholera was only a part.

Ultimately, the salvation agenda focussed on only one of cholera's multiple ontologies, that of public health emergency. The salvation agenda represented a bottom-line agreement to offer necessary and vital palliation in the face of a deadly disease. It is here we see a striking similarity between the 'anti-politics machine' and the salvation agenda insofar as the exigency of saving lives depoliticised cholera and its socio-economic conditions through the operations of a technical, internationalised, ostensibly ethical and apolitical humanitarian apparatus.

Moral Witnessing: Vulnerability, Mortality and Improvising Medicine

The existential stakes of Zimbabwe's political-economic meltdown were made drastically apparent at the clinical sites where cholera was treated. Here, I share stories from healthcare workers, volunteers, journalists and campaigners who witnessed the gruesome effects of the disease and were thus willed into action to help stop the outbreak.

Pastor Tom Deuschle recalled the harrowing scenes at Harare's specialist infectious disease hospital on Beatrice Road when he visited it as part of a missionary outreach project through his church:

> I visited Beatrice Road infectious disease hospital and could not believe what I saw. There were about 300 people outside with drips that were hanging from trees or from the fence. I became angry and indignant, I wanted to know why they were not in the hospital. We went inside the hospital itself. The whole place was covered in vomit and diarrhoea. We had to wear gumboots to walk through the mess, which was several inches deep.

The smell was of blood, vomit, diarrhoea and urine. There were bodies piled on top of bodies, piled on top of bodies. There weren't enough beds, not enough buckets and not enough medicines. In the paediatric ward, we saw four young children. One of them had his eyes rolled into the back of his head. I asked why they weren't on drips and I was told that they only had adult drips and that these kids would be dead in the morning. We saw the mortuary which was just a room with stacks of dead bodies in it. They ran out of body bags and they wrapped children in disposable plastic bags from supermarkets. And the bodies were sliding and falling off each other. I had never seen anything like that. This is no way to run a country and I was pissed off.[6]

Similar scenes were unfolding throughout the country. As MSF travelled around Zimbabwe setting up cholera treatment facilities, the organisation documented experiences of people living with the scourge of cholera and the country's wider health crises. 'We are refugees in our own country,' said Blessing, a young man interviewed in front of Bindura's Chiwaridzo Clinic (Médecins Sans Frontières 2009b). Outside the centre lay seventy-one cholera patients. Left unshielded from the naked rays of a scorching sun, interrupted by periodic torrential rains, these patients were prevented from entering the building – itself a cesspool of diarrhoea and vomitus. The open-air tents where MSF delivered treatment were quickly overcrowded and filthy. On top of this, neither the government nor the patients had any food. The awful conditions at this site, as was the case at many others,[7] diminished the morale of healthcare staff, both foreign and domestic, and rendered humane medical treatment extremely difficult. The inadequacies of 'staff, stuff, space and systems' (Farmer et al. 2013), as described in Chapter 2, added further impetus to improvise the clinical care for the living and to improvise the disposal of the remains of the deceased:

Case management is difficult under the bad conditions of the site. A woman, 50, died a couple of days after MSF arrived in Chiwaridzo, but in the crowded corner none of the staff noticed she was dead until hours later. The deceased was lying among other inert and exhausted cholera victims. The MSF Environmental Health Officers (EHO) had to disinfect and wrap

[6] Tom Deuschle 2015 int.

[7] Interview, Kudakwashe Katurura, Medical Director of Celebration Health, Harare, 10 September 2015.

> the body in front of the other patients; there was nowhere else to do it. 'How can you treat someone like this,' said one of the MSF EHOs. There is no mortuary either in the clinic or, of course, in the camp's field. The body was set to lie in the corner of the camp next to the patients under the boiling sun. There was nowhere else to store it. Eleven hours pass before it is taken away. (Médecins Sans Frontières 2009b)

Accounts from healthcare workers, in my interviews and in public documents, endowed the act of caregiving with a special moral urgency, largely founded on the sense that imminent harm could be avoided, and existing pain could be mitigated, with a concerted humanitarian effort. Pia Engebrigtsen, a Norwegian nurse, worked for two months with MSF in the Masvingo province. For Engebrigtsen, the speed with which cholera kills was critical to shaping her understanding of the nature of the epidemic and what could be done about it. The epidemic was different to any other emergency she had dealt with previously. On entering a new area, she and her team would meet so many people sick from cholera. Their clinics were soon overwhelmed. She knew that, unavoidably, lives would be lost. Death from precipitous dehydration hastened the necessity to make rapid but wise decisions about triage, case management and use of resources, as '[t]omorrow might be too late' (cited in Médecins Sans Frontières 2009b). Furthermore, the extensive spread of the disease meant that MSF was stretched thin, struggling to balance individual care with public need in systematic and consistent fashion. Engebrigtsen went on to describe the devastation of seeing parents who lost their whole families to the disease. She poignantly depicts an image of survivors silently mourning the passing of their loved ones with only their eyes betraying their pain, hopelessness and guilt for not having brought family members to the health facilities earlier. Of course, the Norwegian nurse acknowledges, the barriers to accessing care were legion at that time – 'lack of money, lack of transportation means, lack of knowledge, huge distances' (cited in Médecins Sans Frontières 2009b). Nevertheless, she maintains that international aid, delivered quickly, efficiently and decisively to areas of need, would have spared 'so many more lives'.

An anonymous MSF volunteer blogged about her experience of being in a cholera treatment centre after returning to her home country. She spoke of the entanglement of her own emotions with the feelings of those whom she saw suffering needlessly.

> My feelings were with the little girl lying on the floor with an IV drip in her slender arm, sleeping of exhaustion. They were with the two young men carrying in their stepfather who fell ill after eating a sweet melon from their farm and who fell into shock when they reached the camp. They were with the old man trying to pull the IV drip out of his arm and leave the camp as he had been there for days without eating because of food shortages. They were with the brave smile of a twenty-year old woman, nine months pregnant. They were within sight of the restless doctors and nurses who forget to eat and sleep to keep the patients alive, the ambitious logisticians and helpers who build structures to allow the sick to lie on beds, have a roof above their heads and some dignity in fighting the disease. And my feelings were with the 45 community volunteers who came together in the morning to get information about the disease and instructions on how to prevent infection, which they then carried back with them to their neighbors and friends. (Médecins Sans Frontières 2009f)

Figure 4.1 below is an image from cholera treatment centres.

Just south of the Limpopo River that demarcates the Zimbabwe–South Africa border, thousands of Zimbabweans congregated at

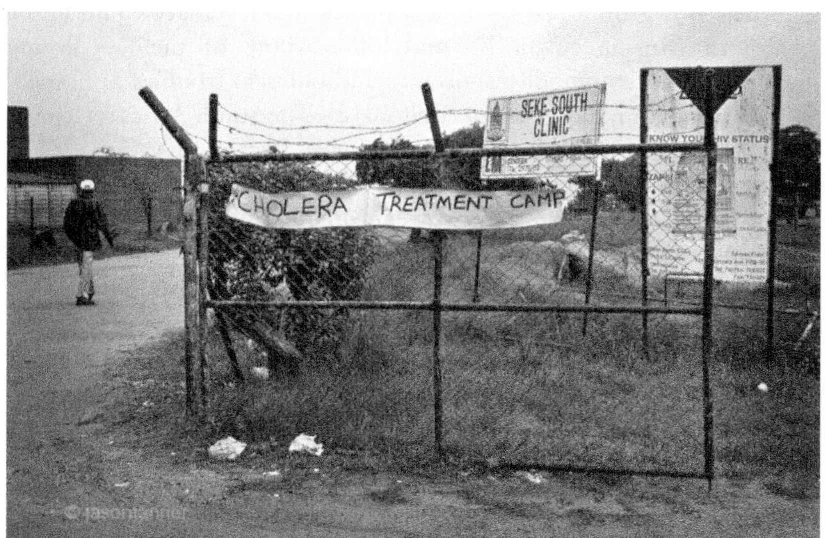

Figure 4.1 Makeshift cholera treatment centre in the high-density suburb of Chitungwiza on the outskirts of Harare.
Source: Jason Tanner Photography

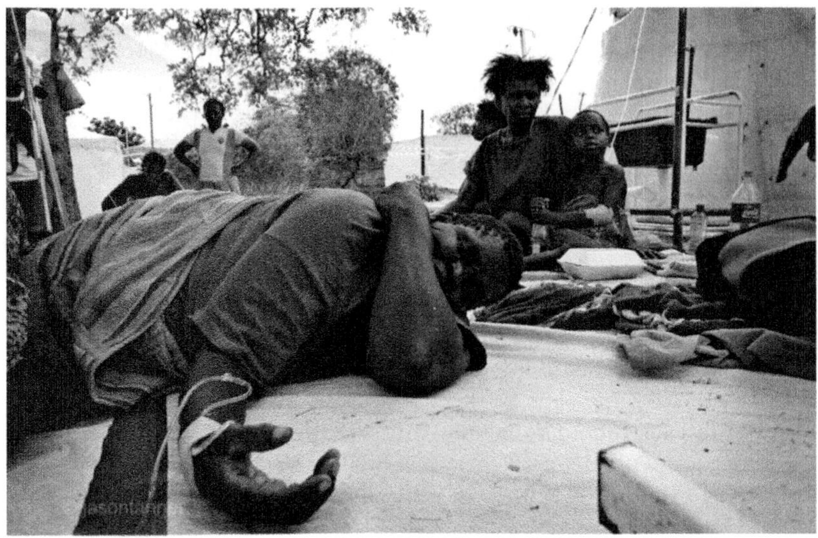

Figure 4.2 Cholera on the South Africa–Zimbabwe border.
Source: Jason Tanner Photography

Musina Showground, an open field turned into a refugee camp in the centre of Musina town, by mid-2008. Many of them – fleeing hyperinflation, commodity shortages and political troubles at home – sought asylum in South Africa (Bolt 2012). The South African Department of Home Affairs opened a Refugee Reception Office at the 'showground' to process claims. However, the South African government considered most Zimbabwean immigrants to be economic migrants and therefore not eligible for refugee status, thus leading to the deportation of large numbers of Zimbabweans before, during and after the cholera outbreak (Edelstein, Heymann and Koser 2014). The bureaucratic processing of asylum claims and possible deportations was slow and often inefficient, leaving Zimbabwean immigrants in the showground for prolonged periods of time and in significant need of basic shelter, water, sanitation, food and health care (Médecins Sans Frontières 2009d).

By November, when the cholera outbreak spilled over from the Zimbabwean border town of Beitbridge into South Africa, the disease easily spread through the crowded living conditions of the Musina 'showground' (Figure 4.2). The South African government soon issued major public health alerts about the epidemic in Limpopo province and mobilised a multi-sectoral response to cholera (Hogan 2008). MSF extended its operations from Zimbabwe to South Africa, screening people at the 'showground' and other sites to identify those with potential signs of cholera for treatment and/or referral to Musina Hospital. The organisation worked in conjunction with the South African government to carry out a wider public health campaign, including hygiene promotion, water and sanitation improvements, and health education activities, in the surrounding area. Much like in Zimbabwe, MSF workers in South Africa recorded testimonies of the hardships endured by cholera sufferers as a result of political crisis and economic collapse in Zimbabwe, as these words from a thirty-three-year-old man staying at a temporary shelter in Musina attest, 'All of us people at the Showground [Musina], we are not here because we want to be. We are here because we were suffering in Zimbabwe. The masses are hungry – they are running from their own country' (quoted in Médecins Sans Frontières 2009d: 7).

Stories of suffering – such as those documented by MSF – were also stories of resilience. The anonymous MSF volunteer mentioned earlier recounts the valiant efforts of the singing staff of a Christian medical charity, the patience and stoicism of cholera sufferers and their family carers, and the ever-expanding team of dedicated volunteers in the community: 'I was filled with encouragement and admiration for everyone working so hard to ease the patients' suffering brought about by an ugly disease which did not have to happen.' In this way, she concludes, 'the sound of cholera' was not reducible to doom, but was also 'the sounds of life that continue despite it all' (Médecins Sans Frontières 2009c).

The above accounts, primarily from MSF workers, are vivid but by no means unique. I gathered similar testimonies from journalists, doctors, nurses, students, civil servants and politicians who stepped into the treatment centres. Through stories of agony and healing, accounts of terrible need and altruistic voluntarism, and reflections on the pain wrought by an ugly and avoidable disease, the treatment centres concentrated collective attention on the critical need to set aside partisan differences, embrace a common sense of purpose, and act on bodies afflicted by or at risk of cholera. In other words, these testimonies speak of the sheer necessity and urgent possibility of salvation: the deliverance from harm, ruin and loss.

The Formation and Politics of 'the C4'

The declaration of the cholera outbreak as a national disaster was a watershed moment in the trajectory of the epidemic. According to a joint report by the Ministry of Health and the World Health Organisation (2011), the declaration led to the establishment of a multi-sectoral task force under the leadership of the Zimbabwe government. The report states that the Ministry of Health 'took the key leadership and coordination role across all stakeholders' including a wide range of government ministries, United Nations agencies, private donors, bilateral government agencies, NGOs and community-based organisations. Meanwhile, the UN Humanitarian 'Cluster' system was activated. Clusters are groups of humanitarian organisations, within and outside of the UN, in each of the main sectors of humanitarian action such as water, health, nutrition and logistics. They are designated by the Inter-Agency Standing Committee, the primary mechanism for inter-agency cooperation in the delivery of humanitarian assistance, and have clear responsibilities for coordination.

To coordinate the responses to Zimbabwe's broad humanitarian crisis, a Health Cluster chaired by WHO, a Water, Sanitation and Hygiene (WASH) Cluster chaired by UNICEF, and a Logistics Cluster chaired by the World Food Programme were all set up. A new entity, the Cholera Command and Control Centre ('the C4'), co-chaired by the Ministry of Health and WHO and directed by Dr Steven Maphosa, was established specifically to coordinate the work of different agencies involved in the cholera response. The C4 also coordinated the inputs of key technical expertise including from the International Centre for Diarrheal Diseases Research from Bangladesh, the American Centers for Disease Control, and the Global Outbreak Alert and Response Network. Resources were mobilised for the work of the C4 and its partners from multiple donors including the African Development Bank, AusAid, the government of Botswana, the Central Emergency Response Fund, the UK's Department for International Development, the European Commission, the government of Greece, the Republic of Korea, the Swedish International Development Agency, USAID and World Vision Australia, among others. The multi-sectoral response was mobilised across several different domains to address the thematic areas of surveillance and laboratory management, clinical case work, WASH, social mobilisation and logistics. Figure 4.3 is a schematic

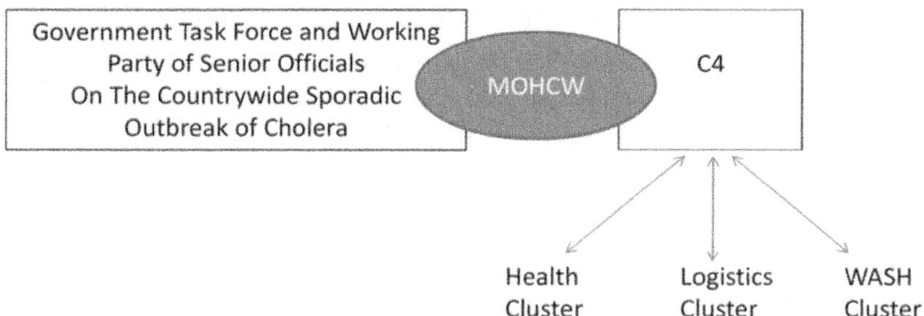

Figure 4.3 Central role of MoHCW in coordinating the multi-sectoral response.
Source: Joint report from WHO and Ministry of Health in Zimbabwe

outline of the organisational structure of these different entities; it shows the central role of the Ministry of Health and Child Welfare (labelled as MoHCW in the diagram) in coordinating the multi-sectoral response.

In reality, the process of coordinating a large-scale humanitarian relief effort was riven with competing claims to leadership, authority and legitimacy within and between different government and non-governmental bodies. The stories I was told about this aspect of the response variably threw blame, self-exculpated, or admitted to personal and institutional failures while almost consistently exhibiting a moral righteousness about saving lives. These stories invoke the salvation agenda, directly or indirectly, to justify bypassing political conflict, including the polemics of 'emergency politics' discussed in the previous chapter, in favour of technically sound and morally imperative intervention.

At the outset, there was intense disagreement over where to locate the C4 geographically in order to host stakeholder meetings. The obvious site, the Ministry of Health offices at Kaguvi House in Harare's central business district, did not allow for round-the-clock access because it is a secure government building and, more importantly, the building itself did not have functional sanitation facilities owing to the urban water shortages. Stanley Midzi, Director of Disease Control and Epidemiology in the Ministry of Health at the time, laughed at how pitiful the situation was when he told me that under normal circumstances a building in the state that Kaguvi House was in should have been closed under the Public Health Act. In this case, however, it was simply too embarrassing for the minister to invoke the act to shut down his own offices.[8] For partner agencies, the irony of a Ministry of Health building being unsafe for meetings because of public health concerns severely undermined their confidence in the government and their willingness to acquiesce to its stewardship. Additionally, staffing in the ministry was erratic, as civil servants and administrators would frequently abscond from work to engage in other business activities to supplement their miserable government salaries. I quote Boniface Nzara, a UNICEF worker, who explained how difficult it was to take the government seriously when its offices were dysfunctional:

> At Kaguvi House, there was no water, there was no electricity, there was nothing! In terms of seriousness, I would say no. Actually, it's a few of them [civil servants] who would commit themselves to government duties. Most of the people were doing any other business like going to their farms. The few who remained, of course, we worked with them very well and they assisted. But government was not serious. Even the statements that they would say on radio – 'we've contained cholera' – we did not take them seriously. Even the communities did not take them seriously. That's why you find that during that time, whenever you went out and asked communities where they are getting assistance, whom they are working with, they would actually say the name of the NGO that is within their area. They would see labels like UNICEF or maybe UN or something like that, and that was the popular pronouncement.[9]

As a compromise, the C4 was eventually situated in the WHO Annexe at Parirenyatwa General Hospital. This meant 'that resources for C4 did not come directly to building capacity in the [Ministry of Health and Child Welfare], [but] it also meant that the centre was able to function at full capacity as quickly and effectively as possible' (World Health Organization/Government of Zimbabwe: Ministry of Health 2011). Despite such neat claims in the post hoc evaluation report, my interviews with practitioners working with and through the C4 suggest a messier picture. Toendepi Kamusuwe, now with Action Aid, was part of the national taskforce against cholera representing civil society organisations. He described the C4 meetings in the following way, 'Government could only provide the buildings and the space but not

[8] Interview, Stanley Midzi, Harare, 22 September 2015.
[9] Interview, Boniface Nzara, Harare, 15 September 2015.

even teas, not even logistical support. ... Then of course in the operations, UNICEF would coordinate the operations.'[10] Itai Rusike, Executive Director of the Community Working Group on Health (an influential local network of approximately thirty-five health-related community-based and civic organisations), and Ben Mbaura of the International Organization for Migration were regular participants in the multi-stakeholder meetings for the humanitarian relief effort. Both told me that the Ministry of Health was so severely under-resourced in terms of materials and workforce that it could not exercise any meaningful leadership over the multitude of international agencies operating in the country.[11] As Rusike claimed,

> I remember in one of the meetings, one of the UN agencies saying, 'we are putting in more money than what is coming from the Ministry of Health in terms of the cholera case so we need to have leadership.' And for sure, they got the leadership. There was no leadership from the ministry in terms of the cholera response. The international [agencies] took over. But because the international [agencies] did not have the experience of working in the community, it was a mess. It was a mess! Cholera came to an end but we can't give credit to the international NGOs. I will not give credit to the international NGOs because most of them, they messed up within the community.[12]

Goldberg Mangwadu, Director of Environmental Health at the Ministry of Health and Child Welfare, expressed similar sentiments, insisting that 'when the donors came in to begin with ... they wanted really to run the show. They wanted really to run the government of Zimbabwe. They started setting their own organisation, their own structures, their own reporting system.'[13] In Portia Manangazira's more even-handed assessment, excellent work was done by all stakeholders but, crucially, she adds that in certain respects, 'all sides were found wanting'.[14] From her perspective, the ministry could only provide 'loose coordination' because of its incapacitation in terms of material resources and its limited available workforce. However, she argued that both the government and the non-governmental partners were equally 'ignorant':

[10] Inteview, Toendepi Kamusuwe, Harare, 23 November 2015.
[11] Interview, Itai Rusike, Harare, 12 October 2015; Interview, Ben Mbaura, Harare, 17 November 2015.
[12] Itai Rusike 2015 int.
[13] Interview, Goldberg Mangwadu, Harare, 17 September 2015.
[14] Portia Manangazira 2015 int.

'You would have people saying they had managed cholera but then it would turn out that it was five cases only.' At the same time, she admitted that partners 'would want to know from the Ministry what we needed and we didn't know! We didn't know whether we needed five tents or 15 beds, and then you get 30 patients, what do you do?' Manangazira asserted that in most instances, 'the partners did a very fantastic job but in some, they added to the chaos'. She told me that certain partners, craving praise, in her view, went 'to international media [to shout] about what they were doing'. And yet, when she confronted such agencies, it turned out that they had been working at field sites in different parts of the country for weeks without knowing how to set up a cholera treatment centre according to national and international protocols. 'That's why I'm saying', she concluded, 'all sides were found wanting.'[15]

When the Government of National Unity was formed and Henry Madzorera assumed the post of Minister of Health, he wrestled with the question of how to work with so many different international partners to avoid conflict and to maintain trust, coordination and unity of purpose. The most important rift, according to many of my informants, between the government and an international institution was with MSF. The strained working relationship between the government and MSF illustrates two very different conceptions of the state. The image of a developmental, bureaucratic state – albeit one in acute crisis – aspired to and held by Zimbabwean civil servants, local NGO workers and many ordinary people jarred with MSF's model of humanitarian rescue. For the former, the cholera crisis signified a profound rupture in a historical trajectory of state-led delivery of public health and authority over non-state actors in the country and it was this rupture that needed to be repaired. By contrast, Peter Redfield (2005: 334) characterises the latter's operational sensibility as follows:

> If MSF perceives a significant crisis in terms of health care in any setting, be it an emergency, such as a cholera outbreak among displaced people, or a policy issue, such as ineffective national malaria protocols, it responds with whatever combination of passionate speech and instrumental action it deems appropriate and can muster. Significantly, this response almost never claims to represent a comprehensive solution or to conform to conventional

[15] Ibid.

utilitarian rationales of public health. The majority of its operational programs justify themselves through moral legitimacy rather than through cost-effectiveness. By demonstrating what is possible, the MSF doctrine suggests, a technically efficient project can highlight the failures of political will behind inadequate health care and remove the excuse that 'it can't be done'. At the same time, members of MSF rarely suggest that their work will directly build a better social order or achieve a state of justice. The goal is to agitate, disrupt, and encourage others to alter the world by practicing humanitarian medicine 'one person at a time'.

The tension between 'the bureaucratic state' and MSF's 'humanitarian rescue' reflects the multiple ontologies of cholera and sharply reveals how different actors, based on their different histories, ideologies and institutional ambitions, acted on the outbreak and clashed while doing so.

Madzorera complained to me that 'some organisations' were uncooperative with the coordination structures that had been put in place: '[S]ome organisations had a mind of their own and left to themselves, they could just go at a tangent. MSF is one such an organisation. They have this great propensity for running their own show in your own country.'[16] Madzorera was astonished when I told that him that an MSF report, published in February 2009, claimed that the organisation had treated approximately 75 per cent of all cholera cases in the first half of the outbreak, a total of 45,000 people. While he mistook the claim to mean that MSF had treated 75 per cent of cholera cases for the full duration of the epidemic, his reaction nevertheless indicates frustration with the organisation and an incredulity at what he saw as a masking of the contribution of other actors and agencies involved in the response:

They're crazy. That was a huge outbreak. We're talking about 100,000 cases. How can they talk about 75%?! MSF operates in specific sites. And they cannot claim to have treated 75% of 100,000 cases. That is mind-boggling. What they're doing now is to undermine the role of other players. We had many, many other players inputting into the system. What I can say is that definitely they did not treat 75% of the cases. They didn't. I can't quantify but they did not treat 75% of the cases. That's what they said?!

[16] Interview, Henry Madzorera, Kadoma, 16 October 2015.

In contrast, several of my interviewees spoke of MSF as both one of the most effective, even if one of the most stubborn, organisations involved in the humanitarian response. Ben Henson, a senior WASH specialist working with UNICEF during the cholera outbreak, noted that 'MSF is notoriously difficult to work with in terms of coordination.'[17] He characterised their modus operandi as both impatient and self-efficacious – 'they simply say "forget all these bloody meetings, we will just implement" and they do a fantastic job.' The C4 meetings were time-capped at one hour to attract and hold the attention of MSF, in particular. As Henson described it, 'if you have rambling three-hour meetings, they will just get frustrated and opt out.' Despite their evident efficacy and extensive management of the cholera outbreak, Itai Rusike excoriated MSF. In his opinion, MSF overstated its contribution and importance to the humanitarian relief effort, concentrated primarily on short-term and emergency measures, sent inexperienced staff into the field, and worked awkwardly with other agencies especially local NGOs:

> MSF, they always have this thing of whenever they go to any crisis, they don't want to see the crisis end. Somehow, I don't know. It's like they survive on crisis, which I think is very unfortunate. I engaged the director then. We had so many meetings with him and we asked, why is it that you think MSF should get all the credit? Us, as local NGOs might not have the kind of resources that MSF has but we played our part and we never ever said, 'this is the percentage of our contribution'. How then do you quantify that? ... MSF has this hit-and-run approach, which we also don't agree with. It's like they are always looking for low-hanging fruits, why? In our engagement with the ministry, we were saying they should have the Rwanda approach where NGOs do not choose where to go. ... At the end of the day, what is it exactly that they were doing? ... To me, Oxfam did a lot more. In all the urban areas, [Oxfam] put up water tanks. They drilled boreholes. And also [German Agro Action]. They did a lot more than what MSF did. MSF were bringing very junior doctors. Very, very junior doctors. I remember going to Beitbridge with Portia [Manangazira] to one of the outreach centres. And we saw a clueless doctor. Completely clueless. They were bringing very junior doctors until they were engaged by the ministry and asked to work with local doctors that were more experienced. So, MSF should not get that credit. They don't deserve it.

[17] Ben Henson 2015 int.

I made numerous and repeated attempts to secure an interview with a representative from MSF who had worked in Zimbabwe during the cholera outbreak. After multiple enquiries with the organisation, I eventually received an e-mail saying, 'unfortunately ... we have to abstain from participating in your study. The issue is still felt as politically charged and participation might therefore affect our current good standing with medical authorities and in prolongation of our current medical activities.'[18] I managed to have a brief face-to-face encounter with a former MSF worker who was Head of Mission for one their branches during the outbreak. She politely declined to give an interview and said that the whole experience was so traumatic that she left not only MSF but all humanitarian and NGO work after the epidemic. Based on my interviews and on the changes in tone in MSF's current commentary on its work in Zimbabwe compared to its previous writing, it would appear that the organisation is now toeing a more cautious line in Zimbabwe after stoking much ire during the cholera outbreak; however, I am unable to verify this beyond conjecture.

Evidently, the institutional responses to the outbreak were permeated by multifaceted disputes and intersecting critiques. How were such differences and oppositions overcome to mount what was ultimately a successful operation in terms of stopping the outbreak? The Ministry of Health and WHO (2011) report states that, 'In spite of the challenges with coordination and the many different perspectives on what needed to be done, all stakeholders were united in a commonality of purpose and a determination to stop the avoidable loss of life from cholera that was afflicting the nation.' Here we see the salvation agenda as the rhetorical driver of action and as justification for bypassing the political in favour of the technical and the ethical. I delved into these issues with Portia Manangazira as I sought to understand her views on if and how the Ministry of Health forged alliances with international and local non-governmental agencies given the divisive politics that I have just delineated. She reinforced the salvation agenda in the following way:

> I remember even talking to some of the partners and saying, 'Look here your government is fighting my government but that doesn't mean that you and I should stop working.' ...you think about the person out there in the rural

[18] MSF Worker (personal communication, 4 November 2015).

area who has lost a child and is about to lose another child. They just want good health for their children. They don't care which government is fighting which government. They want to see their children through school and become adults and live in harmony in the community. They don't care which government is fighting which government. Sometimes, they don't even know which politician is responsible for the country. If people could do much more wherever they are, it'll be a much better world. ... [Humanitarians] should just come and do what they came for and then let the political mechanisms of the world deal with the messy politics that is affecting human health.[19]

Ben Henson explained that UNICEF 'went under the political radar and just worked from a technical perspective with the technicos in the Ministry of Health ... Basically, we ignored the political claptrap. And I don't know whether others have told you similar things.'[20] Many others did in indeed tell me similar things. The views of multiple development organisations working through the C4 are captured by Ajay Paul of German Agro-Action (now Welthungerhilfe) who said,

There wasn't the breathing space to go through the political dimension of this [cholera outbreak], or the accountability mechanism of this. Agencies have got different roles to play and our role certainly wasn't to do anything other than immediate response, life-saving response. We were too busy with that.[21]

Having given some insight into the intricate politics of forming the C4, I shift focus from the dynamics of bureaucratic organisation to the work done in clinics and communities by volunteers who joined the campaign against cholera.

Medical Missionaries

After Pastor Tom Deuschle, Andrew Reid, a consultant physician specialising in HIV medicine, and Kudakwashe Katurura, a junior doctor specialising in surgery, visited Beatrice Road Infectious Diseases Hospital as part of an outreach trip for Celebration Health, the medical programme of Celebration Ministries International, they resolved that something had to be done to end the horrors of cholera. Katurura emphasised to me how this trip etched itself in their minds:

[19] Portia Manangazira 2015 int. [20] Ben Henson 2015 int.
[21] Ajay Paul 2015 int.

Our pastor [Tom] almost broke into tears. He said, 'look guys what can we do?' That night we didn't sleep. The pastor said 'I'm going to call my international friends and partners. You guys put down a proposal so that at least we can take these city council guys back to work.' We put down a proposal. We sent it through. We got a little grant – almost a half million bucks.[22]

What followed was a massive philanthropic drive. In Deuschle's account,[23] he met with Dr Prosper Chonzi, Director of Health Services at the City of Harare, to ask how much money the authorities required to cover the salaries of healthcare professionals so that they could return to work. Deuschle then called prominent Zimbabwean businessmen, Strive Masiyiwa (founder and executive chairman of the diversified international telecommunications group, Econet Wireless), Nigel Chanakira (founder of Kingdom Financial Holdings Limited), and 'several American churches' to help. Channelling philanthropic donations, Celebration Ministries proceeded to pay the salaries of Harare-based doctors and nurses for the months of December, January and February, the peak of the epidemic. Doctors received a per diem of US$90 while nurses were awarded US$45. Both Deuschle and Reid related this story to me with religious zeal and full conviction of the church's moral rightness in taking these unprecedented actions to address the outbreak. To stress how extraordinary this action was, Deuschle insisted that what he was doing may have been 'illegal' – a church, he told me, cannot legally pay the salaries of civil servants though he declined to explain how he was able to do so – but it was absolutely necessary:

It was illegal but we knew that it needed to be done. I said let them throw me in jail if they want to but we can't sit by and watch this suffering. For me, God's laws are higher than human laws. We have a moral code that we need to live by and that supersedes the legal code.[24]

As for Reid, he stressed the role of the church in running the city's health services thereby delivering salvation for the people of Harare:

What happened was Pastor Tom got the money and, essentially, he paid the salaries for City Health of Harare for basically December, January and February. Maybe more months. And that enabled 15,000 lives to be saved.

[22] Interview, Kudakwashe Katurura, Harare, 10 September 2015.
[23] Tom Deuschle 2015 int. [24] Tom Deuschle 2015 int.

Those were the kinds of numbers coming from the City Health section in Harare. Basically, a church ran City Health for three months. I'm telling you things that nobody in the world knew. CNN, BBC didn't know. Obviously, some of these things are very politically sensitive. It would be a tricky thing to say those sorts of things. But, basically, a church ran City Health and it enabled workers to go the cholera camps and do the job.[25]

In addition to raising the money to pay the salaries of doctors and nurses, Celebration Health also put together an extensive health promotion campaign that included a series of nine television programmes about cholera: what the disease is, what symptoms it causes, how to prevent it through basic hygiene measures, and what to do when the disease is contracted. The capstone project of Celebration Health was Operation Outstretched Hand. In Reid's words, 'Operation Outstretched Hand in the cholera epidemic was really like a war situation. It was like a call to young people to war.'[26] The Operation entailed the mass mobilisation of junior doctors, medical students, nurses, pharmacists, logisticians and drivers through the church's network to respond to the outbreak. The team established large cholera treatment centres in Chegutu, Kadoma, and Chinhoyi where they offered clinical care and ran health promotion campaigns in surrounding areas.

In what follows, I describe the experience of working in these settings by drawing heavily on an in-depth interview with Dr Tungamirai Mhuka, known as Tunga – a 22-year-old medical student at the time of the epidemic and now a junior doctor, specialising in internal medicine.[27] Throughout this narrative, I interweave the views of several other of my informants. Though Tunga's account is an individual one, it is situated in a collective experience of coming-of-age for many despondent young people, who had been left feeling idle and redundant during the economic crisis but who rose to the epic challenge of giving life-saving treatment in the most unfavourable of circumstances. In Tunga's narrative, we also see a rupture in his political consciousness. As I reveal below, Tunga's self-professed faith in Zimbabwe's nationalist project, with its claims to liberation and development, were shaken to the core. He was confronted by the vulnerability and suffering brought about by the country's political-economic meltdown

[25] Andrew Reid 2015 int. [26] ibid.
[27] Interview, Tungamirai Mhuka, Harare, 6 September 2015.

in ways previously unimagined. Tunga's story thus illustrates the larger claims of this chapter: where the state, impeded by a political impasse, struggled to transform a dire social situation, the salvation agenda allowed individuals to exercise their agency in the morally compelling work of saving lives.

'The first thing I heard was Budiriro and Chegutu – cholera is there big time,' Tunga began. His studies at the University of Zimbabwe's medical school had been suspended as there was no money to pay the teaching staff and as wards in the public hospitals shut down. The medical profession was seized with discontent over low pay for doctors and poor working conditions in the hospitals. Nevertheless, Tunga's parents forbade him from participating in doctors' strikes against the government as the situation deteriorated and rumours of a cholera outbreak propagated: 'It was basically two weeks of sitting around and hearing all this coming in. Although, there was a suppression of information.' After about three weeks of 'mutterings', it eventually came to light that Zimbabwe was in the throes of a 'big outbreak': 'And that's when we knew that we were in trouble. People knew. By that time, the country was in no position to respond. Fortunately, at that time, there were a lot of NGOs with interest in health that were there.'

One of the NGOs that Tunga was referring to was Celebration Health. The charity had been invited to assist the local council in Chegutu with managing the epic escalation of cases of cholera in the town in late December. Dr Katurura was leading the medical team on the ground along with Dr Reid. Katurura remembered their arrival in Chegutu vividly:

> When we got to Chegutu, oh my goodness! We got there like 4 or 5pm. The danger was. . . the way a cholera camp has to be set up, it has to be: go in, go through the stages, then come out. You don't mix people because they are in different stages of their treatment. But [what we found] was just haphazard: women and men were mixed. People were vomiting. It was horrible. I said, 'look guys, thank you very much but we are taking over.' We began to structure the whole camp from scratch. We set up separate male and female wards. We set up our tents. We had infection control measures. We started setting up everything.[28]

[28] Kudakwashe Katurura 2015 int.

In their first night in Chegutu, after re-designing the cholera treatment centre, the team began to treat patients in conveyor-belt fashion. According to Dr Reid, they 'spent the whole night treating people … there were three nurses who put up 1,000 bags of IV fluids that night. 1,000 litres in one night. What we did as docs, we just banged in cannulas all over the place.' Spirits were invigorated by gospel singing in the twilight hours just before dawn, 'the three sisters, after putting up 1,000 bags of fluid that night, basically started singing … "Rudo raMwari", the love of God. … Then these sisters began weeping and weeping. It was amazing.' Such stories circulated through the church's network, poignantly attesting to the resilience and impact of its volunteers and bearing witness to the vitality of Christian 'Samaritanism'. Tunga, a practising Christian and a member of the Christian Medical Fellowship, was invited to join the efforts of Celebration Health in Chegutu.

On arrival, Tunga was astonished by scenes at the clinics. Patients were dying at a phenomenal rate as the number of cholera cases continued to rise inexorably, compounded by delays in replenishing stocks of the necessary medications, such as antibiotics and intravenous fluid, to treat the sick.

After the camp got set up, it was just an explosion. From late December – I remember I spent New Year's away from home for the first time in my life because normally we do it as a family but this time I was out there in the boondocks, so December/January I was barely home. You'd come back for two weeks and then you go back only to find that it's getting worse and worse and worse. It was just an escalation in December and January. When you go online and see the stats, you're just like, 'What's going on?!' It was really a scary time for us. At the same time, we were excited because we were doing clinical work away from consultants and no one was shouting at us. We were actually working and getting things done. That was exciting but at the same time, we were scared. We were like, 'This is real, this is cholera, this is real!' It was that mixed emotion.

Tunga and other volunteers worked indefatigably. Further assistance came from MSF, and, together the two organisations brought the situation under control in Chegutu. From there, Celebration Health moved on to Kadoma to work in concert with MSF and UNICEF.

One night in early February, Tunga recalls that the number of cases in Kadoma 'exploded from a hundred people to 600 or 700. Overnight! … It exploded from a hundred people to nearly 700 people from between maybe 4pm and the next morning.' The volume of cases exceeded the capacity of the cholera treatment centre set up at the local hospital. They migrated the camp to a larger site, a football pitch right in the middle of the city. The different agencies gelled together and their combined effort 'started making a difference and then the deaths dropped – we reached a point where we were not recording deaths anymore and it became a case of keeping track of who went in and who went out.'

At the same, Sikhanyiso Moyo, an environmental health officer from the Kadoma city council explained to me that while the volunteers like Tunga did extraordinary work in their medical humanitarian response to cholera, they did not have the capacity, nor the mandate, to attend to the fundamental causes of the outbreak, which were to be found in the city's dilapidated hydraulic infrastructure and lack of decent water supply:

> We have some challenges in terms of water supply in the city. We have some areas that haven't received water for the past five years. Now with cholera, it's a waterborne disease. You'd find that it was a great challenge to us. We were spreading the word that people should wash their hands. That people should rehydrate themselves. Whereas we didn't have water in the city. We also had some sewage overflows. They are a common sight in the city. You'd find that it is very difficult to control the diarrhoeal diseases when we've got sewer overflows. We also have the waste heaps all over. We could see that although we were trying to fight the outbreak, we had challenges. To educate someone to improve hygiene practices when you've got sewer overflows and when we do not have the water itself, it was a challenge.[29]

Tunga and I talked extensively about his emotional reactions to the cholera outbreak and to being part of the medical humanitarian response. He, like several others whom I interviewed at Celebration Health, commented on the speed with which the medical charity responded to desperate need. He also stressed the flexibility that Celebration Health exercised in its protocols and practices, especially compared to the sclerotic, cash-strapped government bureaucracies. On a personal level, the responsibility and industriousness demanded of Tunga combined with the remuneration he earned made him feel that he had come of age. Responding to the outbreak marked a transition

[29] Interview, Sikhanyiso Moyo, Kadoma, 17 November 2015.

from being a medical student, who felt acutely cast aside when the country's medical institutions ceased to function, to being a medical humanitarian, a professional caregiver doing the arduous work of saving lives in the midst of a public health nightmare.

> Being paid was a very new concept to us. We were kids. Yes, times were tough, but we were used to asking parents for help. We barely suffered from the long queues in banks because we were still very much dependent. [Celebration Health] offered to pay us per day. They would pay us when we came back from the field. You'd spend a week at home then go back to field. We didn't even really use that money. We used to buy groceries for home, airtime, a pair of jeans and then go back into the field. It was actually quite exciting. We were helping people. As students who were almost finishing their training, we felt relevant. That was another big thing. We actually felt relevant.

At the same time, this coming of age was accompanied by a political awakening. For Tunga, the experience was 'life changing' and it transformed him into 'a different political animal': 'I think from high school, I had always been a conformist. I always went with the system. I followed the rules. By that time, I began to question those in power at a level that I never ever have.' The cholera outbreak raised profound social and political questions for him about justice and inequality. Moreover, it diminished his faith in the country's political system and stirred a new historical consciousness, one critical of ZANU (PF)'s patriotic history and its claims to modernising development.

> I was born and bred ZANU(PF). I am anti-colonial and anti-neo-colonial. I know that Great Britain is wealthy in part because it has plundered countries like ours. Nevertheless, our leadership has failed us. I had supported the farm occupations, in fact, I thought it should have happened much earlier. But when I got to [the University of Zimbabwe], and I got more exposure to what's happening in our country, that's when I began to see the corruption and failure of our leadership. ... We saw the real life of what this cholera outbreak was like. It was pretty scary. It was an eye-opener. ... I used to have a lot of trust in the system. I don't have trust in the system anymore at all because I saw it fail [during the cholera outbreak]. I now started questioning a lot of things that I saw. From that time onwards, it changed what I was. I would no longer blindly follow or blindly believe. I learnt to ask a lot more questions. I also learnt that I deserve better. There was a real shift for me personally at that time. ... Our leadership has failed us. '08 proved that beyond all doubt.

When I asked Tunga what motivated him during the outbreak, he offered a compelling and uplifting story of young people rallied together through the church and the Christian Medical Fellowship to help fellow citizens dying from an appalling disease. When I probed further into the politics of it all, he lamented the internecine blame game that unfolded between the ruling party and its opposition. It distracted the country's elites from urgent matters on the ground and left ordinary Zimbabweans to the deal with the crisis on their own. Indeed, Tunga insisted that to be effective in the cholera response, it was vital to 'turn a deaf ear' to partisan politics and to suppress whatever anger, indignation, fear or regret that he and others felt about the country's crisis:

> We were born into a functional, good country but then there was just a decay, a gradual decay of governance and the economy [that] led to this final scenario we were in. ... People were angry but people were also afraid. Remember we had just come from that '08 election. People were angry but then no one articulated it in that way. There was this fear. There was this fear. People were angry but they stayed quiet and reserved. They didn't voice it out loud. But then there was definite anger. There was a feeling of being let down, especially for the medical students who were unsure of their futures. People were very angry. People were very disappointed. But at the same time, we had a lot to do. In the end, we just ignored that and focused on work at hand and what we had to face and hope that the medical school would be open soon. That's what we ran with.

Finally, I asked him what impact the experience had on his political allegiances having been raised in a staunch ZANU(PF)-supporting household. Capturing a widespread sense of paralysis and political pessimism, he simply responded, 'I am now a spoiled ballot until a decent opposition emerges.'

Tunga's narrative echoes essential aspects of the salvation agenda but it also reveals much more than this and allows us to see the political subjectivities that emerged through the cholera crisis. We see a venting of outrage at the failures of the state under ZANU(PF) – a sentiment that is widely shared as I discuss in Chapter 5. We see a shift in historical consciousness about the country's trajectory in which expectations of the state as the bringer development are suspended but there remains hope that in due course, Zimbabwe will return to being 'a functional, good country'. And we see the creative, moral agency of responding to a crisis for the sake of individual and collective survival.

The Possibilities and Pitfalls of the Salvation Agenda

'One of the great things about Celebration Health,' Andrew Reid proudly declared to me, 'is that it has worked in submission to the Ministry of Health not in opposition. There were no political agendas and that was great because there is a danger that political agendas can destroy people working together.'[30] Reid continued to explain that Celebration Health was so effective because it was part of a coherent, unified programme to treat cholera, working in harmonious concert with local government and other non-state actors. Tom Deuschle made the same argument more vehemently, commending the focussed, high-minded work of Celebration Health and denouncing NGOs and UN agencies from entwining themselves in Zimbabwe's divided politics thereby undercutting their own effectiveness. For him, at least rhetorically, the church has a primary duty toward salvation in all senses of the word and that duty comes before, above, beyond and after politics:

> I won't talk about the politics of that outbreak. Things were very divided at that time and I'm not interested in who was saying what. We did our work under the radar and we let the politicians take the credit ... The church is more important than any government – in fact the church is its own government and it has been here for more than 2,000 years. African governments change like changing underwear compared to the longevity of the church. And the church will still be here when ZANU and MDC have gone. You may think that I'm anti-government from what I've said. I'm not. I'm anti-corruption and I don't care who is responsible for it. I pray for my government and I pray that our leaders don't seek office for personal enrichment. But it is wrong for churches to get involved in party politics. We sit outside and above political parties in our organisation, in our moral code and in the interests we serve. We were well received in the communities in which we worked because people trusted the church; we were not caught up in the politics like the way the NGOs were. The UN agencies did a lot of work but they were slow and bureaucratic. They weren't able to move quickly on the ground like we were. All those organisations came into full effect when we had already been running cholera camps for two to three months.[31]

[30] Andrew Reid 2015 int. [31] Tom Deuschle 2015 int.

Undoubtedly, Celebration Health's contribution to the humanitarian relief effort was profound. Through a combination of budgetary support for clinicians' salaries and direct medical intervention, the charity estimates that it was responsible for treating 30,000 people during the outbreak. It is impossible to verify the accuracy of these figures, which are inherently difficult to evaluate owing to the poorly functioning health information systems at the time and the multi-stakeholder nature of responses at treatment centres and in the community. Nevertheless, it was clear from my interviews with local and national government figures that Celebration Health – along with MSF, Merlin and UNICEF – played an indispensable medical humanitarian role during the epidemic.[32] Organisations such as the Red Cross, Oxfam, German Agro-Action and the World Food Programme, among several others, were essential to the broader public health programmes, particularly in the WASH sector, nutrition programmes and health education. All these measures were the programmatic arms of the salvation agenda.

Nevertheless, medical acts leave a political trace (Abu-Sada 2012). For all that communities welcomed the largesse of the international relief effort, questions emerged about the more fundamental aspects of socio-economic inequality that undergirded the outbreak; I discuss some of these in more depth in the next chapter. Humanitarians themselves were sharply aware of their limitations in this regard. Joanna Stavropoulou, a communications officer with MSF, described visiting the high-density suburb of Dzivarasekwa where she and her mobile team were running a WASH programme in the community, primarily injecting a concentrated solution of chlorine into containers of water to ensure that it was safe to drink (Médecins Sans Frontières 2009g). The team also treated local water sources with chlorine. 'Why can't you fix the whole urban water system?' a man asked the MSF team. Another resident joined the conversation asking, 'Is it for life, is it forever this treatment you are doing?' Stavropoulou explained to them that MSF is an emergency organisation that was there to help with the cholera epidemic. After this exchange, the resident who posed the questions refused to have her water chlorinated. Stavropoulou then asked the resident if she was afraid that she would fall sick without

[32] Interviews with Portia Manangazira (Ministry of Health), Stanley Midzi (Ministry of Health), Steven Maphosa (WHO), Madzudzo Pawadyira (Ministry of Local Government) and Sikhanyiso Moyo (Kadoma City Council).

chemically treated water. The woman quipped in retort, 'But then when you stop giving this, we will be affected even more than before.' An eavesdropper chimed in, adding that, 'We are resistant like wild dogs; we've been drinking unsafe water for a long time.'

Further illustrating the tension between emergency intervention and long-term development, the Red Cross insisted that its prerogative was to save lives by offering technical solutions to Zimbabwe's water crisis. The organisation assisted in the rehabilitation of waterworks in Chegutu and Kadoma. When unable to fix underlying, chronic infrastructural damage, the organisation focussed on enabling access to other clean water sources such as water tanks and boreholes. This was explained to me by Abel Gumbo, the health and social services coordinator for the Zimbabwe Red Cross Society. I probed further, asking him about the political dimensions of the cholera crisis and the limitations of narrowly focussed technical interventions. He was candid in saying that for the Red Cross engaging with the country's politics would present a stumbling block to the organisation's work:

> To us, I think that is too political. As Red Cross, we don't look at all those things. We look at saving lives and helping people where there is a problem. But the background to what is happening, we don't usually want to hear that. Otherwise it disturbs our work. We would not be able to function if we look at all those things.[33]

I challenged Gumbo, pushing the argument that 'if you don't look at all those things', then it is difficult to be effective, especially since political decisions and economic mismanagement dovetailed with social inequality to give rise to the urban water crisis. Gumbo remained adamant in his position, firmly stating that 'looking at politics will not solve anything especially for Red Cross.' He then went on to typify the Red Cross's response to complex emergencies as fire-fighting without interrogating 'where the fire has come from, you know' because 'you don't want to be looking at that kind of thing otherwise you will not exist. Us, we are apolitical so whatever happens: people are fighting, we don't take sides. We just look at our mandate.'[34]

For James Munyaradzi, a resident of Chitungwiza and local NGO worker who had been involved in aspects of the cholera response, the humanitarian relief came to something of an abrupt end, foregoing

[33] Interview, Abel Gumbo, Harare, 17 August 2015. [34] Ibid.

more long-term rehabilitation and development work, especially in the high-density areas of Harare: 'Once it was under control, the clinics cleared and everybody went home. … A few guys then stayed behind and did a few more boreholes. But it was like: Thank goodness, it's over, now we can all go home and rest.'[35]

The salvation agenda ultimately achieved its aim: it galvanised a disparate array of actors and institutions to save tens of thousands of people from ruin, harm or loss because of cholera. As I have argued in this section and throughout this chapter, it did so by ignoring the complex multiple ontologies of the cholera outbreak in terms of its historical and political-economic determinants and dimensions, and focussing collective attention and pooled resources on urgent need that warranted immediate action. The salvation agenda was not without its pitfalls. Most obviously, humanitarian relief came at the expense of longer-term action. As Miriam Ticktin (2011: 63) has framed it, critics of humanitarian action argue that in the absence of other types of long-term structural responses coordinated or enacted by political movements, or even by institutions like the state, humanitarian and disaster NGOs end up filling in the gaps resulting in the conservative management of social and political problems, 'one that works to retain what is already there, rather than to change it or to plan for a different future'. This is a consequence of favouring the technical over the political in the cholera epidemic insofar as the technical response was geared toward the specificities of the temporary administration of medical relief and the mitigation of a lack of clean, potable water in vulnerable communities.

A related problem emanated from the tension between moral witnessing and political engagement. Organisations involved in the response, who had been working in Zimbabwe since before the outbreak, knew the risks of speaking out against the government. They faced de-registration, deportation and possible prohibition from working in the country again. Brian Patrick, a humanitarian worker with a major international organisation that has done several missions in Zimbabwe and has a long-term in-country presence, discussed with me the calculus that NGOs have to make under such circumstances:

[35] James Munyaradzi 2015 int.

What I would say is that there is trade-off that agencies have to make sometimes between speaking out about things and getting the job done. And I think that in doing that they are making a calculation; the calculation is 'can we help more people by being present here and doing the work that we are doing or by speaking out about what's happening and challenging it?' I think that because they are operational organisations not really advocacy organisations – although many of these organisations also do advocacy – there tends to be, at least at the programme level, bias in favour of maintaining the operational presence of their work and recognising that the impact of getting kicked out of the country can be very long term. If you get kicked out of the country, you can be kicked out for five to 10 years. You might not get to go back in the foreseeable future. There is, if you like, a bias particularly on the part of the local programme to stay present rather than to speak out.[36]

Patrick elaborated explaining that in the early 2000s, his agency became aware of a cholera outbreak in northern Zimbabwe but chose not to publicise it. Instead, the agency opted to provide emergency relief in an apolitical fashion. They used neutral descriptions of the situations they encountered rather than politically loaded ones. For instance, they deliberately explained food insecurity and malnutrition in terms of drought and environmental change rather than politically motivated restrictions in access to food, and they deliberately avoided use of the word 'famine'. Similarly, they avoided the word 'cholera' for fear of its political connotations and instead spoke of 'acute watery diarrhoea'. He justified the decision as follows:

And I suppose my question, which I don't pretend to have the answer to, is would we have had a better response to the cholera outbreak, that saved lives and prevented the spread of cholera, if my agency had spoken out about it? My gut feeling is no, but I don't pretend that is authoritative and I recognise that I don't have access to all the relevant information. What I think would have happened is that the government would have shut us down, not cooperated with us, probably shut down other agencies as well. I don't just consider my agency getting shut down, I consider my peers getting shut down too. There is peer pressure.[37]

Such are the real-world politics of humanitarian relief.

By now it should be abundantly clear that the complexity of Zimbabwe's political crisis and the intractable, historically produced predisposing and precipitating factors that led to the outbreak could

[36] Interview, Brian Patrick, London, 6 July 2015. [37] Ibid.

not be resolved or rectified through the delivery of life-saving treatment alone. At the same time, there was no collective drive on the part of humanitarians to deal with the epidemic's underlying determinants. Given the diversity of institutions involved in the response, each expressing wide-ranging views on the true origins of, and allocation of culpability for, the cholera crisis; each asserting different claims to legitimacy in response to the disaster; each restricted by its operational mandate and its access to donor funds; and each accountable to different constituencies, it is little wonder that it was the salvation agenda which prevailed as the primary response. To paraphrase Albert Camus (1967) yet again, the salvation agenda is what had to be done in the never-ending fight against disease and its relentless onslaughts, despite their political disagreements, by all who, while unable to transform the system but refusing to bow down to pestilences, strive their utmost to be healers.

Conclusion

I began this chapter by sharing testimonies of harrowing scenes at the cholera treatment centres. I argued that witnessing the spine-chilling clinical and social effects of cholera ignited the moral imagination of medical professionals, relief workers, development specialists, religious volunteers and bureaucrats to forge a diverse alliance dedicated to saving the lives of those afflicted by cholera and to remove the most proximal causes of the disease. The motivating impulse behind this alliance was to address the force majeure of the dysfunctional Zimbabwean state through what I have called the salvation agenda, itself a powerful moral and rhetorical force. The salvation agenda allowed agencies and actors to set aside their multiple, interlocking disputes over the causes of the epidemic and responsibility for its resolution and to focus instead on averting imminent death.

Like Ferguson's anti-politics machine, the salvation agenda presented a complex political, socio-economic reality as a defined problem amenable to technical fixes. Thus, it is unsurprising that when the outbreak passed, 'it was like, thank goodness, it's over, now we can all go home and rest'.[38] Crucially, unlike the anti-politics machine, the salvation agenda did not expand Zimbabwe's bureaucratic state

[38] James Munyaradzi 2015 int.

power. To the contrary, the assemblage of institutions involved in the medical humanitarian response treated the cholera outbreak primarily as an emergency, and they have left behind them an under-resourced and politically divided state that is still struggling to manage the deeply embedded patterns of socio-economic inequality and partisan conflict that initially led to the epidemic in the first place.

In the subsequent and final empirical chapter of this project, I examine how the residents of Harare's high-density townships, which were epicentres of the disease, experienced and interpreted the epidemic in relation to the country's wider social, political and economic dynamics.

5 'People Were Dying Like Flies'
The Social Contours of Cholera in Harare's High-Density Townships

In every phase and aspect of a disaster – causes, vulnerability, preparedness, results and response, and reconstruction – the contours of disaster and the difference between who lives and who dies is to a greater or lesser extent a social calculus.

—Neil Smith, *There's No Such Thing as a Natural Disaster*, 2006

Like any other disease, cholera has in itself no meaning: it is only a micro-organism. It acquires meaning and significance from its human contexts, from the ways it infiltrates the lives of the people, from the reactions it provokes, and from the manner in which it gives expression to cultural and political values.

—David Arnold, *Cholera and Colonialism in British India*, 1986

Despite political attempts to contain, manage, foreclose and define the meanings attached to the cholera epidemic, the disease and the events surrounding it nevertheless acquired a social life of their own. As further testament to the multiple ontologies of cholera, in the aftermath of the outbreak, what has emerged are multiple, complex and often contradictory understandings of cholera and its attendant questions of origins, suffering, body counts, rescue, relief and rehabilitation. Thus, my investigations into the social contours of cholera in the townships reveal ongoing processes of meaning-making through which people grasp and come to terms with the epidemic as a 'man-made' disaster. In Zimbabwe's divided political environment, this involves polarised claims about what really happened and about who the heroes and villains of the outbreak were (cf. Venugopal and Yasir 2017).

This chapter focusses on the views of residents in the townships where the epidemic first fulminated. I examine the stories that township residents told to ascertain how cholera has been committed to historical memory and to see what political subjectivities have emerged from the outbreak. For the clear majority of my informants, the outbreak aroused public anger and outrage at the government for its causal role in the epidemic and in the inadequacy of its relief efforts. However, this anger has not translated into any effective political mobilisation or permanent change. What I show, therefore, is the sense of both political indignation and impotence that cholera has left in its wake. I argue that cholera has embedded itself into historical consciousness as many crises at the same time: a health crisis, a political-economic crisis and a social crisis as well as a crisis of expectations, history and social identity. From here, I make a threefold argument about the political subjectivities born out of the cholera outbreak and its aftermath.

My interlocutors recounted stories of relentless suffering, violence, dispossession and abandonment during the epidemic (a politics of disposability). It is tempting to read this grim narration as a form of victimhood – the surrender of agency – when faced with a sinister political regime. But to do so, I argue, would be to grasp only one aspect of what are layered public narratives. From a seeming position of 'victimhood' my interlocutors launch a muscular, in fact devastating, critique of political power as exercised by the ZANU(PF) government. They unambiguously vent their outrage at the failures of the government to provide welfare and protection for all its citizens. In so doing, they forcefully assert their claims to political status, social recognition and belonging as rights-bearing members of the nation-state (a politics of expectation). Finally, I argue that despite their sense of abandonment by the state – a politics of disposability – and despite their claims to substantive citizenship from the state – a politics of expectation – townships residents also exhibit a remarkable politics of adaptation in how they negotiated and survived the cholera crisis.

The chapter is organised around three storytelling, or narrative, frames – political context, political aetiologies and political responses – through which my interlocutors discussed the cholera outbreak and through which I demonstrate their political subjectivities. I excavated narratives of cholera via in-depth interviews and focus-group discussions with seventy-six residents of the high-density areas of Budiriro, Glen Norah, Glen View, Dzivarasekwa, Kuwadzana, Mabvuku-Tafara, Norton and Chitungwiza. These areas were all terribly affected by cholera. I also conducted a focus-group discussion in Hopley Farm, a poor settlement on the outskirts of Harare, which was not badly affected by the disease. All these interviews were buttressed by a range of more informal conversations, particularly with my 'gatekeepers' – a local taxi driver, Amos; an unemployed but well-educated sanitation specialist in Budiriro, Favor; and a women's rights activist, Winnet Shamuyarira, who is affiliated with the local NGO Katswe Sistahood and works primarily in the townships. What my interlocutors have in common is that they all reside in the high-density areas or, in a minority of cases, have spent a significant part of their lives there even if they have since moved elsewhere. Despite this commonality, the people who inform this chapter do not constitute a homogenous group. Their demographic profile is highly varied. In terms of age, I made an effort to interview across generations and have captured the voices of people who were school children during the outbreak as well as the voices of grandparents who have been in the townships since before independence. In terms of socio-economic status, I spoke to many who work in the informal sector as well as people employed as teachers in local schools and others who have secured jobs with NGOs or the media in the city proper but still live in the townships. In terms of political party affiliation, the overwhelming majority of people I spoke to were hostile to the ruling party even if not outwardly aligned to any of the opposition.

Political Context: 'Everything Made Everything Else Very Difficult'

I began all of my interviews in the townships with the same question: 'What was life like for you in 2008?' My first interviewee, Tsitsi, a sixty-two-year-old resident of Kuwadzana who works as a masseuse, spoke to me in candid detail about this period:

> We suffered in 2008. In general, life wasn't very good at all in terms of contaminated water. City council couldn't afford to buy chemicals. We were drinking contaminated water, which affected us with cholera. So, people were dying like flies. They were taken to Beatrice Infectious Disease hospital. They were being treated there. Some of them survived. But mostly kids and elderly died. When they died, you were not allowed to take the corpse at home like our tradition says we should. The corpse would be wrapped in a plastic bag and buried. And we were not allowed to touch it.[1]

[1] Tsitsi 2015 int.

Tsitsi emphasised the deplorable state of the water supply in the townships. Most of the time, she explained, the taps ran completely dry, but on rare occasions when liquid did come out, it often emitted a pungent smell and bore visible traces of human waste. In her own words, 'in 2008, if you opened the water, it was so dirty that you could see even the shit coming out of the taps.'[2] In thinking back to this period, Tsitsi bemoaned not only the poor water supply but also the lack of food, money and jobs. For Tsitsi and many others working in the informal sector like her, the economic disaster had an inescapably despondent character: it meant more queues, more vending, more begging, more stealing, more sex work and more desperate faces, all interspersed by occasional fits of prayer, reminiscence, rage and alcohol-fuelled bravado (Jones 2010b).

In his ethnography of the dormitory town of Chitungwiza, the anthropologist Jeremy Jones (2010b) investigates the social implications of and responses to Zimbabwe's economic collapse. He describes the economic action that 'ordinary people' – those navigating the urban informal sector with limited recourse to political patronage or foreign capital – resort to as *kukiya-kiya*, a chiShona term that connotes 'cleverness, dodging, and the exploitation of whatever resources are at hand, all with an eye to self-sustenance' (Jones 2010b: 386). Importantly, he argues that new kinds of subjectivity emerge as people adapt in creative, but short-term, ways to economic disaster:

> The result is a radical reorientation to the economy, and consequently a radical reorientation of the economy. Crucial in that regard is the emergence of a generalised culture of evasion: evasion of social institutions like the state, the bureaucracy, and the law; and evasion of cultural norms and hierarchies. In the words of one young practitioner, *kukiya-kiya* is all about a 'zigzag' search for opportunity in the hardened face of reality. (Jones 2010b: 287)

Jones's observations were born out in my own explorations of this period. Before my interlocutors would speak about cholera, they stressed the multiple and profound ways in which the collapsed economy had affected their daily lives. Hyperinflation embedded uncertainty into all quotidian activities from travelling into town to grocery shopping, from looking for work to caring for the sick:

[2] Ibid.

We had a currency that you could not call a currency. You go into town for $1.2 billion bus fare but then coming back, you need $3 billion. The amounts were exorbitant, they were meaningless in any case. ... Someone did not have money and would spend two days queuing at the bank. We used to leave home at twelve midnight to wait for the bank which opens at 8 am. After spending eight hours in the queue and getting a little money, the amount of money that you would have got would not be enough to purchase a loaf of bread by the time you leave the bank. It was the scenario of money being in very high denominations but was useless – just printed papers. That even affected schools because some children need bus fare to come to school. But the bus companies, the combies, did not have enough fuel and so they would hike the prices up according to how much he has been charged for a five-litre can of diesel. So, it was not safe going to work if you were a commuting public: you should have three times the amount you pay in the morning. If you are told that it costs a million to get into town, then you need to have another three million on standby.[3]

The desperation and uncertainty of this period saw many young women turning to transactional sex work to secure their livelihoods and look after their children. In focus group discussions I was told that since Operation *Murambatsvina*, a shift in social norms and economic activity had taken place. Transactional sex epitomised the short-term time horizons in which people were thinking and acting. I met with a large group of sex workers, convened by my gatekeeper from Katswe Sistahood, Winnet Shamuyarira, in Hopley Farm to discuss the conditions of 2008 and the cholera outbreak. This group of women had previously resided in different high-density townships in the south-western flanks of the city but had been moved to Hopley Farm during the operation. One woman described the shift in social norms and the rise of sex work as follows:

What we noticed is that when we moved to [Hopley Farm], it doesn't matter that maybe this is her husband or this is my man, we just exchange. For today, I have to go to him because he has $3 but tomorrow I go to someone else because he has $5. We just exchange. It was very sexy! [applause and roaring laughter from the group] When you're taking our history, it seems as if it's a joke. But it was very real, you couldn't laugh. At the time, we did it and you were given cash. You could then feed your family; we don't even think of kids to go to school. Nothing like that. You can only think of feeding the kids. So, by the time, we would even thank god because we could

[3] Interview, Samuel Muchero, Glen Norah, 2 September 2015.

feed our kids through the sex exchanges. We don't even bother with dressing them. We don't even go to buy clothes. We just think about the food. And it wasn't protected sex.

The short-termism of sex work as described above, as well as many other forms of *kukiya-kiya*, can be understood in terms of Achille Mbembe and Janet Roitman's (1995) notion of 'stupor'. This stupor represents a violent departure from the ways things used to be and admits of no normal solution. In other words, Zimbabweans, like the Cameroonians who are the subject of Mbembe and Roitman's paper, can no longer plan their lives or make decisions, and, more profoundly, that the country is no longer part of the evolution of history (Mbembe and Roitman 1995). What is most pertinent here is Jones's argument that the adaptive logic of *kukiya-kiya* became the dominant and ostensibly most necessary response to the crisis. He delineates a reinforcing feedback loop in which short-term economic activity is 'deployed in response to a historical predicament that is itself mired in the short-term' (Jones 2010b: 298). Moreover, he argues that the 'very bureaucratic institutions that were supposed to lay the ground for "straight" progress have themselves been operating in *kukiya-kiya* mode' (Jones 2010b: 298).

The logic of *kukiya-kiya* in Zimbabwe's bureaucracies was amplified by the broader political context of the country's fiercely contested presidential and parliamentary elections of 2008. The mass informalisation of the economy was politicised in that it was bound up with socio-economic and institutional networks and relations of patronage (Alexander and Chitofiri 2010). In the townships, where the opposition MDC members were marginalised, ZANU(PF) affiliates could access state resources through political favour. In this way, my interviewees asserted that food supplies to the townships – whether commercial or humanitarian – were often siphoned off and redistributed among politicians, councillors, party activists or agents of the state, such as police and soldiers. To quote a focus group participant in Dzivarasekwa,

[T]here was mealie meal that was coming from Zambia. When that mealie meal became available in the shop, it created problems, chaos and violence. You would be in the queue for four or five days without accessing the mealie meal, there would be chaos and then the soldiers would come under the guise of bringing some sort of order. But they were doing it so they could beat people and buy the mealie meal instead of anyone else. ... Some of them would then sell the mealie meal back to us on the black market, and they were making plenty of money.[4]

Put another way by Paida, a young woman living in Norton, 'The poor remains the poor. Even when the food came, those people on the higher, they get the food. People on the ground, they don't get it.'[5]

Such dynamics not only compounded the widespread food insecurity and hunger in the townships; they augmented deep political divisions and fuelled widespread suspicion of ZANU(PF) as a nefarious party that had co-opted the state and was determined to use its machinery to make life difficult for the urban poor – many of whom sided with the opposition in 2008 and earlier. Further still, the political violence of this period occasioned a 'rupture in social norms' (Alexander and Chitofiri 2010: 674). Jocelyn Alexander and Kudakwashe Chitofiri (2010) argue that this violence rendered neighbours and family relations 'unknowable', thereby reconfiguring social, familial and other inter-personal relations in township communities. As one of my interviewees attested, walking within her neighbourhood became terrifying in 2008 'not because of robbers but because of the opposition party [and] the ruling party', since, at any time, she could be stopped unexpectedly and asked to produce her party membership card: '[W]hich card am I supposed to produce because I don't know who is asking – is this guy from opposition or from ruling party? ... People have been raped when they found that you don't have the right card.'[6]

As noted earlier, an important consequence of the battle between ZANU(PF) and MDC was the undermining of urban governance (McGregor 2013). The intense political struggles that occurred in local councils were visible to township residents and were seen as anathema to professional service delivery and harmful to the lives of ordinary people. According to an elderly man in Budiriro,

The main problem lies with this political wrestling between MDC city council members and ZANU(PF) city council members. At the end of the day it is the grass that suffers when these elephants fight. At times, you find that when the MDC councillors want to provide good services, the ZANU (PF) councillors want to tarnish their image by saying that they are not doing anything. So, there's this infighting in the council. It's affecting service

[4] Focus Group Discussion, Dzivarasekwa, 7 October 2015. [5] Paida 2015 int.
[6] Interview, Chipo, Hopley Farm, 23 September 2015.

delivery. It's not that resources are not there; they are there. The money is there to buy [water treatment] chemicals but only this infighting between the councils is causing the problems. We can't manage our own things, we Africans. Fighting for political muscle is the problem. … These are things causing problems, especially in areas perceived to be MDC strongholds. If the councillor for this ward is MDC, then they isolate you as well in terms of service delivery. That's also a problem.[7]

The result was a profound lack of service delivery and social cohesion in many township communities. The violence and hunger created a toxic synergy that compounded the cholera outbreak. And importantly, among my informants, a deep resentment toward ZANU(PF) was solidified. To quote Samuel Muchero, a primary school teacher in Glen View,

What was worse was that the political field was so polarised. There was so much political violence prior to the outbreak of the disease. We had people running away from their rural homes because of the political violence. By the time they came here, they thought there was safety here but then there was an outbreak here. Everything made everything else very difficult. The politics of the day was what mattered most. It was that which created this monster. If the politics was stable and people were going to work, I think that outbreak would have been managed much earlier and deaths could have been prevented.[8]

Political Aetiologies: 'The Government Is the One Who Caused the Cholera'

As cholera ravaged Harare's high-density areas, many Zimbabweans watched with concern, then disbelief and eventually horror as scores of people succumbed to infection. In the first three months of the outbreak, before it was declared a national disaster, the Ministry of Health promoted individual health behaviours to curtail the spread of cholera – extolling the virtues of good hygiene such as hand washing, drinking clean water, eating hot food and so forth. This was their desperate strategy for explaining and addressing the outbreak. Amanda Chikaura, a Harare-based journalist, investigated the outbreak from its

[7] Interview, Elderly man, Budiriro, 17 September 2015.
[8] Samuel Muchero 2015 int.

early stages tracking the official response to it and the reception of public health messages in the townships:

> The whole epidemic was caught in the crux of the elections. You need to locate what you're doing within the political-economic milieu of 2008. It was the year of elections. It was the year of the harmonised elections and then the run-off. And there is a history of how resources that should have been going to public services were being diverted towards campaigning. At no point did we ever stop to think about the human lives. I think I stopped counting when I got to 18 – 18 deaths! – because I was like this cannot be happening in Harare in the 21st century without someone being held to account. There was no support for families in terms of let's help you bury your loved ones, let's help you have a funeral, let's help you understand what happened, let's help you understand that this death did not occur because you were unhygienic. And that was the dominant message that the state sent out was that you're becoming diseased a) because of sanctions and b) because you're dirty. And I think it is such a dangerous message for black people to be given. It is denigrating, it is dehumanising and of what I know of the township life – because part of my life has been spent in the township – people in townships are extremely hygienic to the best of their means. And they are quite fastidious about cleaning up their own garbage. What was happening was that council wasn't collecting refuse, water wasn't flowing and so there was a contamination of faeces in drinking water because families had to dig wells in their backyards and when you shit where you live – I have no other way of saying that – your water table is going to become contaminated with bacteria and excrement. It became a disease that affected people on a particular side of the railway tracks. And the final narrative that I picked up was that you're getting sick because you voted for the MDC and this is punishment.[9]

According to James Munyaradzi, a resident of Chitungwiza, the view of the urban poor as 'filthy' circulated widely among the elite and middle classes, who were largely divorced from the local realities in high-density suburbs. As he said to me in exasperation, 'You would hear people saying things like, "why don't [the urban poor] just wash their hands?" And you're trying to explain that they don't have any water and then people ask why they don't have any water.'[10] As such, the dominant narratives in the media and public health messaging around cholera obfuscated the structural factors that precipitated and propagated the disease. Such narratives marked graduated forms of

[9] Interview, Amanda Chikaura, Harare, 2 September 2015.
[10] James Munyaradzi 2015 int.

citizenship. They distinguished individuals and communities who possess 'modern medical understandings of the body, health, and illness, practicing hygiene' (Briggs and Mantini-Briggs 2004: 9) – sanitary citizens, to use Briggs's terminology – from other individuals and communities, such as township residents, 'who are judged to be incapable of adopting this modern medical relationship to the body, hygiene, illness, and healing – or who refuse to do so' and thereby become unsanitary subjects (Briggs and Mantini-Briggs 2004: 9). In this schema, the latter are seen as less deserving of substantive citizenship rights through access to public services and must take individual responsibility for their poor hygiene or else suffer from cholera.

In the townships, however, the themes highlighted in Chikaura's statement above – the deaths of citizens from a preventable and treatable disease without official accountability, the government evading responsibility for the outbreak, poor public service provision, blaming and denigrating the poor for their illness – recurred repeatedly across almost all my discussions. When residents were instructed to change their individual behaviours to curtail the transmission of cholera, they were quick to identify the immediate drivers of the outbreak as structural, specifically the collapsing water and sanitation infrastructure and the ever-expanding squalor in their neighbourhoods. Moreover, the analysis of my informants ran deeper. They recognised that the delivery of clean and potable water, the collection of refuse, and the provision of medical care entail an extraordinary chain of human and non-human actors that links them, as township residents and more broadly as citizens, to wider political structures. This chain includes the state, local government, Morton Jaffray waterworks, engineers, electricity supplies, water treatment chemicals, doctors, nurses, food supply systems, medicines and so forth.[11] Residents were thus aware of their vulnerability at every step where links in this chain might be missing or broken. But most importantly, my informants stressed that the functioning of this chain – or networks of chains – comes down, as it so often does, to politics.

Samuel Muchero described the cholera outbreak as the result of a 'total breakdown of service delivery' in which the city council was unable to provide water or to attend to the high numbers of burst

[11] Multiple interviews with township residents.

sewage pipes around the townships. Importantly, Muchero blamed the Zimbabwe National Water Authority (ZINWA) for this failure:

There was no water. Nobody looked after the sewer. Unlike in low density areas where you have your own systems and access to water tanks. Here it is something that is communal and it is the responsibility of the council. But because the government wanted to disempower the opposition-led council, the water and sewer was removed from the council and they created a department that they call ZINWA ... which did not have the facilities nor the technical know-how of running those things unlike the council. If people think there was someone who caused the disease, well maybe. I wouldn't think it was anybody in particular, it was the result of a total breakdown of services.[12]

This was the prevailing view among my informants regarding ZINWA. Its takeover of Harare's water management was widely understood to have been a cynical political move to wrestle public service delivery away from the MDC-run municipality and provide ZANU(PF) with yet another source of public money to embezzle. ZINWA soon earned a reputation for incompetence and was popularly re-branded as Zimbabwe No Water Available. Favor, a young unemployed sanitation specialist in Budiriro, went further and speculated that ZINWA was not simply incompetent but thoroughly corrupt:

If you look at most of the parastatals, there is no productive business going on there. Apparently, there is a lot of looting in most of the parastatals. Look at National Railways of Zimbabwe, look at ZINWA itself – it is a very important arm that is supposed to deliver in terms of water and sanitation but apparently, there is nothing. They were supposed to be revamping the infrastructure ... if ever they are getting money from the Ministry of Finance, they are actually misusing that money. You look at the absurd salaries that are given to top executives in those parastatals, you'd be surprised because somebody is earning $30,000 USD per month or even more [laughs] and yet there is no money for simple purification treatments, chlorine for instance, to purify water for most of the poor people in the high-density suburbs. ZINWA is worse off! And there is lack of accountability when you look at the situation with ZINWA. There was accountability when municipality was taking responsibility of such issues because there is a residents' association and the municipality is answerable to the residents' association. Now

[12] Samuel Muchero 2015 int.

ZINWA is not accountable to that particular organisation. It's a corruption. It's a non-performing entity. It's a white elephant, as it were.[13]

Favor's diatribe against ZINWA is perhaps less important for the veracity of the claims he makes – although investigations by NGOs into corruption in parastatals confirm such exorbitant monthly salaries (see, for example, Muchichwa 2016) – but rather for the frustration he unleashes about an institution that has completely betrayed its mandate of water delivery. Moreover, as far as Favor is concerned, this is no straightforward dereliction of duty. For him, Zimbabwe's once rule-bound and expert bureaucracies have self-cannibalised through institutionalised political greed that emanates from the highest ministerial levels and trickles down to even the most local forms of government. This greed enriches those with access to power and leaves the poor to wallow in their own shit, literally.

These views are not held by Favor alone but are, in fact, commonplace in the high-density areas. Tsitsi complained that cholera was a consequence of the corruption of the city councillors, who were 'busy putting money in their pockets instead of buying the chemicals to put in the water'.[14] She also indicted Morton Jaffray waterworks for working in collusion with the city council to set the water rates and then steal that money:

Our main water is by Morton Jaffray. They had no money. They were telling people that they have to pay so much, so that the council can afford to buy chemicals to put into the water but it was a lie. That was the main thing, which killed many Zimbabweans. They were putting money in their pocket.[15]

Favor's mother-in-law, also lamenting the state of the city's water supply, put it thus:

[L]ook at it this way: if you have the power to give me water and you give me dirty water, I would say that you are killing me. That is what was happening. The officials were saying that you should eat a proper diet, good food, but then there was that issue of money. If you didn't have money then you couldn't get food. It wasn't a solution to a problem.[16]

[13] Interview, Favor, Budiriro, 10 August 2015. [14] Tsitsi 2015 int. [15] Ibid.
[16] Interview, Resident, Budiriro, 10 August 2015.

Through the commentaries recounted above, we see political subjectivities emerging from the cholera outbreak, especially the venting of outrage at the cruelty and callousness of a state willing, as they see it, to cause harm to them as unwanted members of the body politic. This is evident in the 'political aetiologies' (Hamdy 2008) that my informants formulate when they extend the pain and misery of the cholera outbreak beyond the pathological organ to implicate a pathological government guilty of, they contend, corrupting state institutions, polluting the public water supply, mismanaging household and environmental waste, and providing inadequate or unsafe food. In the words of several of my informants, 'the government is the one who caused the cholera.'[17] While some believed the government caused the cholera outbreak through the malign neglect of the townships, others literally believe that government deliberately caused the cholera outbreak through the use of chemical or biological agents. I attend to these accusations in more depth in the following sections.

Political Response: 'They No Longer Care about the People'

The implacable ruthlessness of cholera left behind a spectacle of death. The bodies of its victims – the friends, lovers, family and neighbours of my informants – laid bare the political and class fault lines that marked the difference between those seen to have full citizenship rights and those who felt they had been excommunicated from the sphere of political concern. Throughout Samuel Muchero's community, and those of all my township informants, cholera made its presence felt in every aspect of social life. People were afraid to gather in public places; funerals were deserted; trading diminished; and clinics were stretched to capacity. Schools, for example, were terribly affected. The primary schools of Glen View and Budiriro lacked clean water, medicines, sufficient food, and electricity. Such conditions endangered the well-being of pupils and staff alike. Tragically, at Muchero's school, three children died of cholera while an additional thirty-five of them lost both parents to the disease. For this latter group, Muchero lamented how their futures were now precarious and uncertain without anyone to pay their school fees or to look after them. He had given up on any expectation of help from the government and was also frustrated

[17] Multiple interviews with township residents.

by the limited and intermittent support offered by NGOs. I probed further, asking what it felt like to be a teacher in this situation:

> It was really bad for us. Because, we also felt that we were not safe. How do you handle a kid when they start vomiting? Suppose I assist the child, won't I contract the disease as well? It was very difficult. It was also difficult managing the classes. In fact, I would say [that] in October 2008, when we had our Grade 7 examinations, we had to ask for assistance from our local clinics where we had a nurse on standby in case anything happens whilst this child is writing his or her exams. I think from the 16th of November, schools virtually closed. Not that the term had come to end nor was there an official announcement of closing schools but there were no kids coming as a result of parents fearing for their children. Some parents took their children to their rural homes where they felt it was a bit safe. Some parents took their children across the borders. So, virtually we had one-quarter class or one-half class. And in the end, very few pupils were coming to school. Schools were almost closed because there was fear.[18]

Adding insult to injury, the government equivocated about what action to take in response to the outbreak. As Chapter 3 has already shown, there was a systematic drive within parts of the government to downplay the true extent of the outbreak, to suppress information about cholera's course through the country, and to insist that the situation was being ameliorated when in fact the disease was wreaking more and more devastation. What many people in my own middle-class social milieu understood as incompetence or failed national leadership was construed as something deeper and more systemic by township residents. For the latter, cholera revealed that the state – corrupted by the ruling party, undermined by political infighting and crippled by economic mismanagement – no longer provided welfare or protection for the urban poor. As Chido, a teenage girl in Budiriro, said,

> There was no time to buy coffins, no need to buy food for the funeral and no one cried because everyone was very close to death, people died every minute ... [and yet the government] said that there is no cholera [in Zimbabwe] ... [why?] because they wanted people to suffer.[19]

Chido remarked on the futility of tears: she lost her father, her neighbour, her friend and others in quick succession and, after all, she

[18] Samuel Muchero 2015 int.
[19] Interview, Chido, Dzivarasekwa, 14 August 2015.

lamented, 'How can you spend the whole day crying?'[20] Others, meanwhile, noted how the spread of cholera exhibited a domino effect with households surrendering to the disease in a seemingly stepwise pattern, and thus fear, uncertainty and mistrust spread in a similarly aggressive fashion: 'It was like cholera was moving from household to household. You would hear that on this line, six people died today. Then the next day, the next line. Then the day after, the line after. It was like dominoes.'[21]

All the while that this disaster was unfolding, the government had still not declared it as such, further fuelling the belief that townships residents were being malignly neglected. James Munyaradzi describes this vividly in his recollection of the scenes in Chitungwiza:

> There's a clinic in Unit L in Chitungwiza, which is a designated cholera centre. You used to go there and you would actually see tents – rows of tents outside – where people were coming in. We didn't really document it but from what you could see, the number of people who were carrying bodies out of the centre was quite high. We would receive reports, pretty much on a daily basis, that somebody had died or several people were dying every day . . . I used to write for a website . . . I remember I did a story once where I said that the number of people who were dying, according to statistics that were coming out, was the equivalent of about three bus crashes a day. When you have a bus crash in this country, it's declared an emergency, if say 15 to 20 people die. It's an emergency and the government comes in to assist. We got to a point where we were having about the equivalent of three bus crashes a day with everybody dying but it was not declared emergency. This cholera outbreak was not declared an emergency until very late in the day.[22]

On top of this, the government's obstructionism towards the international humanitarian relief effort was apparent to township residents. Chido recalls that the 'whites were not allowed in clinics because of their political ties',[23] and she specifically mentioned that international NGOs were often denied space to operate when they arrived in local communities. The phrase that I heard most commonly when I asked people why they thought that there had been such a delayed and ineffective response to cholera by the government was 'havasisina basa nevanhu' ('they no longer care about the people'). Many of my informants insisted that the state had been transformed into a punishing

[20] Ibid. [21] Glen Norah 2015 FGD. [22] James Munyaradzi 2015 int.
[23] Chido 2015 int.

institution intent on treating township residents not as citizens but as a dispensable population to be managed, politically exploited, beaten into submission or made to disappear according to the whims of the ruling party:

In 2008, we had no food, no money, no running water, no fuel. It was hard to live. We were forced into *pungwes*[24] three times a day and there was a lot of violence. There was a war in this country. The elections were sabotaged in the opposition areas such as Harare, Gweru and Bulawayo. That's why the water tanks were filled with fake chemicals. On top of that, there were no qualified doctors to treat us, only the Cubans who do not even speak our language. How can they understand what is wrong if they can't speak the way we do? They [ZANU-PF] don't care about us because we are Hararians and we are people of the opposition. They are sabotaging people, that's where the disease [cholera] came from. They succeeded in killing us. It was so pitiful.[25]

The government desperately tried to deflect attention away from its complicity in the cholera outbreak, as discussed at length in Chapter 3. The familiar cry of sanctions was loudly chanted as an explanation for the government's diminished capacity to respond to the needs of its people. In the most extreme utterance of shifting the blame, the Minister of Information, Sikhanyiso Ndlovu, declared in mid-December 2008 that cholera was racist, terrorist and biological warfare launched by the British to infringe upon Zimbabwean sovereignty. My informants read such statements with cynical incredulity. Chipo, a sex worker in Hopley, said to me:

We would have to go back and ask what actually leads the government to have those sanctions? You see. What actually leads you to have those sanctions? That's how I can pose my question to them. The sanctions come because there is something which had happened. So, they can't hide and blame the sanctions. How did the sanctions come? How were we surviving before the sanctions? And why do you destroy that relationship that we used to have before the sanctions? We were on the ground. We were the ones who experienced that [cholera]. If the government had to come to stay in Hopley,

[24] During Zimbabwe's liberation struggle, *pungwes* were all-night gatherings, featuring a music gala, in which ZANU drew support for the guerrilla fighters. In the post-2000 crisis, the ruling party reincarnated the practice for whipping up political support at election time. Their association with the liberation struggle further adds to Chido's sense that the country was at war.

[25] Informal discussion with residents of Glen Norah Extension C, 14 August 2015.

would they like it? … When they flush their toilets, when they have water from the tap, when they're enjoying their life – I don't think they would like the way we stay here.[26]

The Zimbabwean rumour mill, a productive machine at the best of times, was running in overdrive as people speculated about the government's role in the cholera outbreak. Certainly, a number of people dismissed outright the suggestion that the British caused cholera in Zimbabwe. Tsitsi would not entertain the thought: 'How can the British come here and do those kinds of funny things when we, Zimbabweans, can't afford to buy the chemicals whilst we're putting the money in our pockets? The British have got nothing to do with this.'[27] And Paida pointed out how tiresome ZANU(PF)'s political rhetoric had become, especially where it comes to blaming the foreigners for internal problems: 'But they say all the disease, the British are causing it. Not only cholera. Most of the disease, they say are caused by the British.'[28] Importantly, many of my other interlocutors insisted that it was the ZANU(PF) regime, rather than 'the British', that had launched 'biological warfare' in the country. They suggested that cholera was 'sprayed' into the townships. How else to explain the speed with which it spread and killed? As one focus-group participant in Glen Norah asked, 'If it's just an ordinary disease then how did it travel so fast and so far? … It was like it was moving systematically. We say they put something in our water.'[29] Such speculation was inevitably shrouded in some mystery and confusion. The patterns of the disease and the differences between who lived and who died were seen by some as entirely systematic and by others as arbitrary.

What is salient, though, was a consistent and deep suspicion of the ZANU(PF) government even if clear-cut evidence to make this case could not be produced. Indeed, as Luise White (2000) has argued, individuals speak from social worlds. Thus, the importance of rumours and gossip lies less in their truthfulness than in their intensity, their pervasiveness and their reflection of what is socially conceivable. In this respect, my informants asserted that the same government that had demolished homes and businesses during Operation *Murambatsvina*, the same government that had propagated political violence in the townships, and the same government that had denied people

[26] Chipo 2015 int. [27] Tsitsi 2015 int. [28] Paida 2015 int.
[29] FGD, Glen Norah, 7 October 2015.

humanitarian food aid was surely capable of poisoning water supplies with cholera. As many saw it, cholera was deployed as a means of emptying the streets and thereby neutralising a possible eruption of public discontent at worsening economic hardships; some thought it was a form of punishment against urban opposition supporters; while others claimed that cholera was a tool to precipitate dramatic demographic change to ease the burden on public service delivery.[30]

A generalised sense of disenchantment with existing political channels and processes ran through multiple interviews and focus-group discussions. Many people said that they had simply given up on government for the time being and were turning to alternative sources of welfare and social services, particularly those provided by transnational or non-governmental entities. During the outbreak, it was institutions like UNICEF, MSF, IOM and German Agro-Action that were seen to save the day through the salvation agenda:

> [W]e were introduced to know about the cholera cases by German Agro Action. That organisation came here and we were trained as health promoters, volunteers. So, there were ORPs [oral rehydration points] where people would get help. The ORP was outside the clinic. They pitched tents outside the clinic. Those people with cholera used to go to those tents to get help. That ORP water was being provided. There was transport for those who were severely dehydrated. They were fetched from here to the hospitals by that organisation.[31]
>
> We didn't have water that was coming from our taps. UNICEF came and sunk some boreholes in the community.[32]
>
> Since people were helpless, they were actually relieved to receive help from people from outside. And they were feeling that the government was being negligent. In fact, the government should take care of its own people but when people are coming from outside to help that definitely means that there is lack of responsibility proper.[33]
>
> You are the father of the house but food is coming from the neighbours. Your kids will be angry obviously.[34]

When I asked what role the councils had played in responding to the outbreak, one of the focus-group participants in Glen Norah quickly retorted: 'Was the council still alive?'[35] James Munyaradzi explained

[30] Multiple interviews. [31] Interview, Audrey, Hopley, 23 September 2015.
[32] FGD, Glen Norah, 7 October 2015. [33] Favor 2015 int.
[34] Amos 2015 int. [35] Glen Norah 2015 FGD.

to me the extent to which the government had lost credibility in many of the townships. He captured popular sentiment most accurately when he told me, '[N]ot because of the cholera alone but especially in areas where there was cholera, people do not trust the state. They don't believe in it.' And then he added that when government officials 'come and say they want to start a project in the townships, the general sentiment is just disinterest. People don't care anymore.'[36]

In Hopley Farm, my informants believed that the reason that the cholera outbreak did not affect them greatly was that their vulnerability had been mitigated by the presence of multiple transnational organisations in their community. Hopley Farm, they explained, had been identified as a highly impoverished area after large numbers of people were relocated to live there following Operation *Murambatsvina*. This designation gave license to development and humanitarian organisations to set up an institutional presence in the township. As a focus-group participant explained, 'By the time cholera had started to spread, we already had many organisations working here and helping us. . . . Inter-Country People's Aid had setup cabin toilets here. . . . MSF provided clean, treated water as well as medication. There were many organisations here.'[37] While another FGD participant concluded, 'Here in Hopley . . . we don't deal with the government; we deal with NGOs.'[38]

However, as I suggested in the previous chapter, many township residents did not view the salvation agenda as an entirely legitimate substitute for the state. Residents mounted critiques of the salvation agenda's short-term, emergency orientation. Furthermore, township residents observed that NGOs introduced new and contested social hierarchies, as the parameters of access to and exclusion from social welfare and medical treatment were perceived by many as informal, ill-defined and propped up by highly unequal power relations. An elucidatory example would be access to food aid. In Dzivarasekwa, residents spoke of how certain NGOs would only give food packages based on anthropometric criteria, in this case defined by a mid-upper arm circumference measured below a certain length after adjustment for sex and age, 'They said you had to be 20cm or less at the upper arm. So, if you were more than 20cm then you didn't deserve food.'[39]

[36] James Munyaradzi 2015 int. [37] FGD, Hopley Farm, 23 September 2015.
[38] Ibid. [39] Dzivarasekwa 2015 FGD.

As Tom Scott-Smith (2015: 923) warns, anthropometry suppresses subjective experiences of hunger, thereby rendering 'the starving voiceless, as hunger becomes determined by experts bearing measuring instruments, examining bodies while leaving individuals mute. Rather than talking to people and understanding personal circumstances, such as diets, income and livelihoods, anthropometry reduces people to their bodies.' Similarly, in Glen Norah, residents noted that people diagnosed with HIV had greater access to food through donor-funded programmes, and so several people in this area went to clinics hoping to test positively for the virus.

The notion that the government caused cholera and the mixed reception of the salvation agenda alert us to how the cholera outbreak marked a crisis of historical consciousness and a rupture in normative expectations of the state among township residents. This is captured by the repeated refrain that the government *no longer* cares about the people. Township residents vigorously questioned the nationalist narrative of liberation and sovereignty – so central to ZANU(PF)'s construction of 'patriotic history' (Ranger 2004; Tendi 2010) – which, in the context of the crisis, was popularly read as a diversion from dealing with the most pressing issues in the country. For instance, Gamu, a teenage girl in Glen Norah, complained that politicians in the ZANU(PF) government 'talk about the colonial times but those times passed long back. Even then if you worked for the white people they gave you everything you needed, they understand someone's problems. Our politicians don't understand our problems.'[40] Similarly, a focus-group participant in Dzivarasekwa expressed her frustration with Zimbabwe's post-colonial trajectory when she said, 'I would rather be banned from walking on First Street and keep my dignity than live in a free Zimbabwe without water.'[41] These and other references to more effective public service delivery under colonial rule are hardly nostalgia for the Rhodesian era but are indictments of the post-colonial government's track record and a rejection of its claim to legitimacy as a bringer of 'unity, development and nationalism' (Dorman 2016).

[40] Interview, Gamu, Glen Norah, 14 August 2015.

[41] FGD, Dzivarasekwa, 7 October 2015; the reference to being banned from First Street is an allusion to pass laws and curfews during Rhodesian rule.

At the start of my fieldwork, I drove around the high-density areas and into the town of Chitungwiza with Amos, a local taxi driver acting as an informal tour guide and giving me a geographic overview of where cholera was most prevalent. Throughout the tour, he offered a running commentary expressing disgust at how Zimbabweans have become accustomed to living in squalor; bemoaning the poor conditions of the roads, the ubiquitous open sewers and the piling up of garbage on the pavements; and charging that the 'refusal to provide public services' on the part of the state stems from a combination of a lack of interest in 'MDC areas' and attempts to 'punish people for voting the wrong way.' For Amos, all that we observed on our drive runs counter to any conception of Zimbabwe as modernising and progressing, or as he put it, 'Everything used to be orderly but now it is chaos. Where did it all go wrong in this country?'[42]

This anti-teleological or counter-linear conception and experience of socio-economic change in Zimbabwe is reflected in Jones's (2010b) ethnographic writing. Jones puts forth the idea that the economic, political and social crisis in Zimbabwe bred a moral and technical ambiguity in the 'system', one that undermined the practice and *telos* of both national and personal development. Since the onset of the crisis, Jones writes, a sense of 'frantic stasis' suffused popular imaginaries of the macro-history of Zimbabwe's march to modernity and of the micro-practices of everyday conduct in professional spheres and in the informal economy. By 2008, Zimbabwe appeared devoid of progress. In contrast to the 1980s and 1990s, during which there was a popular expectation of politically driven development, ordinary people and indeed the larger economic and political system had now come to focus primarily on 'making do' and 'getting by' because of the 'current situation'. In the popular imagination, therefore, the cholera outbreak became emblematic of both the malicious capabilities of the ZANU (PF) regime and the sense of historical rupture in the country's trajectory as a whole. In other words, cholera can be read through my informants' narratives as a health crisis, a political-economic crisis and a social crisis as well as a crisis of expectations, history and social identity.

[42] Amos 2015 int.

Between Citizen and Subject: 'Requesting Permission to Arrest All Cholera Sufferers'

In 2008 and 2009, my informants had little choice but to watch those around them dying from human waste. As I have argued throughout this chapter, township residents understood their own vulnerability and the death of those around them in the contexts of dilapidated water and sanitation infrastructure, a weak national public health response, and the arrival of multiple humanitarian actors seeking to stand in where the Zimbabwean government had failed. Through such experiences, many of my interlocutors noted that they were not only afflicted by waste but saw themselves as waste. Much like the human waste produced by cholera, they were superfluous to, unwanted by and expelled from the body politic; their lives and livelihoods were rendered utterly disposable. Tendai Biti asserted that Zimbabwe's 'rogue state' had turned many citizens into objects and articulated his analysis as follows:

> Where you've got a combination of collapse of the state in the sense of the state not being able to carry out its obligations like provision of housing, clean water, electricity and so forth, which is the situation now and was the situation in the meltdown years then you've got on one hand, the collapse of the state, and then on the other, you've got the existence of the predatory state that is beating up its citizens. The combination of the rogue state that has also failed isolates the citizen, alienates the citizen, reifies the citizen, it makes the citizen an object. This feeling. If you feel it in Mbare or Budiriro, you'll feel it even more in Matabeleland. You'll feel it even more in Matabeleland. Again, it is very physical, very visceral. The people become objects. The people become officious bystanders in processes that involve them but exclude them, processes that make them victims but processes that exclude them. That has been the story of Zimbabwe and all autocratic regimes.[43]

This sense of feeling disposable – what I am calling the politics of disposability (Giroux 2006) – captures how township residents felt that they were not only left to fend for themselves in the face of this catastrophic outbreak but were also supposed to do it without being seen by the dominant society (Giroux 2006). The Zimbabwean cartoonist, Tony Namate, illustrated this visually with a satirical drawing that appeared in the UK national newspaper, *The Guardian*. The

[43] Tendai Biti 2015 int.

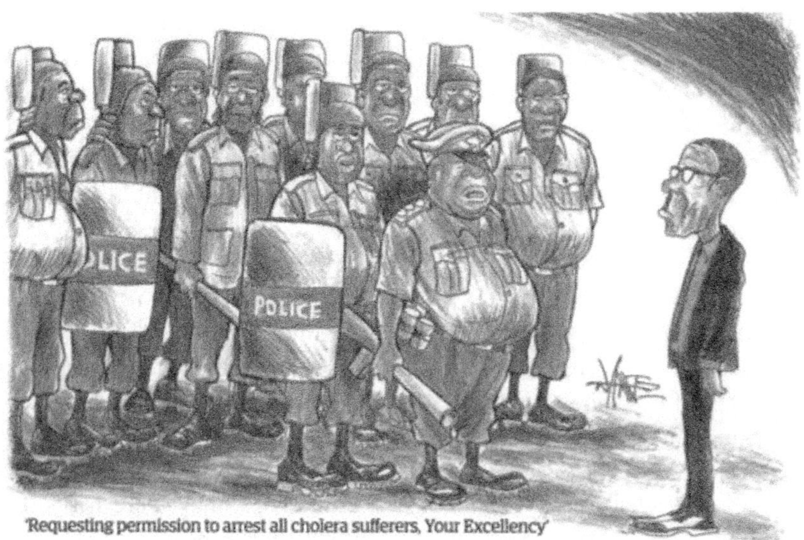

Figure 5.1 Tony Namate's satirical cartoon of a police commander requesting permission from President Robert Mugabe to arrest all cholera sufferers.
Source: The Guardian

image depicts a paunchy anti-riot police commander requesting permission from President Robert Mugabe to arrest all cholera sufferers (see Figure 5.1). The cholera victims' principal crime, it seems, was that they made a socially and politically embarrassing disaster visible to the nation and to the outside world. Of course, the rhetoric of punishment that my informants used time and again suggests that their 'crime' was deeper than that – they were 'guilty' of voting the 'wrong way'. The cholera outbreak and its consequent politics of disposability therefore reinforce the arguments made in the 'sociology of disasters' literature (e.g. de Waal 1997; Guggenheim 2014; Rubenstein 2015; Venugopal and Yasir 2017) that disasters often accentuate the social struggles in a society and underscore the inherent inequities within a political system.

In terms of the politics of storytelling, the testimonies given by my informants sit in contrast with the literature on vernacular modes of critique. James Scott's (1985) influential *Weapons of the Weak: Everyday Forms of Peasant Resistance* is a compelling look at how 'folk descriptions', particularly stories and personal accounts of social relationships, offer a much more visceral and palpable critique of power than does ideological or political discourse. Scott argues further that 'folk descriptions' entail differences between public speech, what he calls 'on-stage performances' or 'partial transcripts', which is sanitised and deferential, and private conversation, what he calls 'off-stage' discussion or 'full transcripts', which is more candid and critical. In an analogous way, a range of scholars writing about disease and healing in Africa have argued that vernacular discourses – that are constructed around the themes of witchcraft and the occult, spiritual healing, heterodox science and traditional religion (Yamba 1997; Schoffeleers 1999; Fassin 2007a; Awah and Phillimore 2008) – about the causes and remedies for epidemics contain within them a moral critique of undesirable social changes and unjust power imbalances in political life.

In the political subjectivities described in this chapter, the critiques of political power were often raw and unfiltered. They were not subtly contained in a vernacular register. This can partly be accounted for by the nature of my interlocutors. The sex workers, for instance, are a bold group of activists who have been asserting their public presence and railing against interlocking systems of oppression that operate in their lives. Through Katswe Sistahood they have adopted a cosmopolitan feminist vocabulary and adapted it to their local circumstances to speak out against patriarchy in its communal and institutional forms in Zimbabwe. It is thus no surprise that, as activists, they were unafraid to air their views.

Along similar lines, many of the people who agreed to interviews were those prepared to vent their grievances. The timing of my interviews is salient in this respect. Memory, Sarah Nuttall (1998) reminds us, is always as much about the present as it is about the past; and therefore the stories told in this chapter were as much about the past as they were about working out what constitutes justice, resistance, freedom, place and survival in the present. Conducted in 2015, two years after the dissolution of the Government of National Unity that had stabilised the economy post-2008, my interviews reflected a moment of declining optimism and increasing fear in Zimbabwe's political history. My interlocutors spoke of a brief reprieve from the crisis during the five years of joint rule between the major parties. However, they had since become much more downbeat about the country's and their own prospects. At the time of interviewing, the cholera outbreak, and the wider politics of 2008, were (re)cast as not only the nadir of the country's contemporary history but as a referent point for how badly the situation could deteriorate. The spectre of 2008 loomed large in 2015 with ever-increasing fear that the country was sliding back into economic collapse, political turbulence, food insecurity and water shortages. Their rage during the interviews cannot be easily separated from the contemporary circumstances in which they were speaking. This therefore suggests that the cholera disaster has not proven to be a 'moment of reinvention', but rather a 'moment of reproduction' in which cholera has both reinforced pre-existing and created new forms and patterns of inequality.

It would be a mistake, however, to conclude that in making such forceful political critiques, my informants all shared the same ideas of where precisely to locate blame, or that they agreed about what it takes to restore Zimbabwe to the path of progress. For many of them, the state, the ruling party, the opposition, the national government and the local government are not monolithic, homogenous entities. While some discussants were dismissive of all and sundry when talking about Zimbabwe's myriad political failures, many others drew astute distinctions between different individual politicians, different institutional bodies such as the much scorned ZINWA and the pitied Ministry of Health, different generations within political parties and different arms of local councils.

I last met with Tsitsi over a cup of Rooibos tea in my office in Harare. During an informal conversation, I let slip my disgust at how our government had (mis)managed the cholera crisis. She burst into laughter, a full and guttural mirth. She insisted that, despite the ordeals she has endured, she would continue to support Mugabe until, as she put it, 'death do us apart'.[44] For her, the freedom that came at Zimbabwe's independence was an act of possession, hard-earned, patient and imbued with historical agency. Mugabe was the vanguard of liberation. According to Tsitsi, the country had not been waylaid by him or other liberation veterans of ZANU(PF), but rather by an unnamed cadre of younger and greedier ministers who did not share the national consciousness born of struggle:

> In terms of looking after its people, ZANU(PF) was very good. In the case of these ministers, these thieves, they are the ones who have ruined ZANU(PF).

[44] Tsitsi 2015 int.

Mugabe himself is a very good leader, for sure he is! And he remains forever and ever. That's our Mugabe and I'll support him 'til death do us apart. It's the ministers in there, weevils so many weevils. They want to get rich![45]

For Tsitsi, cholera was a reminder of the price of freedom and the need for ZANU(PF) to keep pursuing its historical mission of emancipation and prosperity for all Zimbabweans. Hers is a politics of expectation and an understanding of citizenship as universal belonging within the body politic. Nevertheless, Tsitsi hastened to add that her view belongs to that of a particular generation. She sighed as she told me that 'these young ones', the 'bornfrees', 'have found [only] hardship in this Mugabe's regime and they don't want to know about him'.[46] For them, Tsitsi acknowledges, cholera was an especially bad episode in a litany of catastrophes that has afflicted the country over the last several years. Favor, who remains unemployed in his mid-thirties despite his qualifications and much needed skills as a water, hygiene and sanitation specialist, looks at the country's truncated horizons for youth as the political abandonment of a generation: '[I]t's like Zimbabweans are surviving on auto-pilot, there is no government.'[47] My talkative interlocutors in Glen Norah, Gamu and Chido, offered a bleak prognosis for the future. When I asked them what they thought about the prospects of change and progress in the country now that the cholera outbreak had passed, I was told: 'I think Zimbabwe needs to copy the revolution in Libya. We were born in poverty, we live in poverty and we will die in poverty.'[48] Finally, for my interlocutors in Glen Norah, the cholera outbreak was testament to their individual resilience and ability to withstand the vagaries of Zimbabwe's crisis:

We didn't have energy to be angry. Everyone was like trying to find a way to survive. So yes, we were angry but it's like, 'what can you do with your anger?' Most of our energy was focused on survival . . . With everything that happened that year, it taught us perseverance. Yes, it was a bad year. For us who survived, it taught us perseverance and it also taught us that there is a god. We didn't survive because we are clever or we are intelligent but I think it's by the grace of god that we survived. It brought out a strong Zimbabwean. From all that experience we became a strong people because we know

[45] Ibid.; the use of weevils in this quote is a local idiom for people in positions of power who abuse their authority for personal gain and take advantage of those beneath them.

[46] Ibid. [47] Favor 2015 int. [48] Chido 2015 int.

that we can survive anything. That year we should have died but because we survived, we now know that we can survive anything.[49]

Neither citizens in the expansive and substantive versions of the concept nor subjects deprived of political voices and rights, my informants tell stories that reveal a relentless tension in their political subjectivities and historical consciousness between a politics of disposability, a politics of expectation and a politics of adaptation.

Conclusion

This chapter has offered an account of the lived experience – the social contours – of the cholera disaster in Harare's high-density areas. By looking at the narratives of my informants, I have demonstrated how deeply politicised the outbreak was in every phase and aspect of its unfolding from the broad social conditions of its emergence (political context) to the immediate circumstances that precipitated it (political aetiologies) and finally to the action taken, or not taken, to address it (political responses).

Recent studies of urban politics in Zimbabwe have explored the continuities and the dramatic shifts in state–society relations heralded by the country's post-2000 crisis. Studies of Operation *Murambatsvina* (Potts 2006b; Fontein 2009) have argued that the state's demolition exercises reveal its arbitrary and spectacular power thinly veiled under appeals to creating urban order. As a consequence, the urban poor recognise the language of the state in terms of its claims to orderliness, but they experience the state, through its use of military and police force, as violent and capable of destroying lives and livelihoods on a whim. The electoral violence of 2008 brought about a rupture in social relations, rendering friends and neighbours 'unknowable' as communities were torn apart by partisan loyalties (Alexander and Chitofiri 2010). The collapse of the economy directed many Zimbabweans into a broad variety of short-term strategies for survival through all manner of street hustling (Jones 2010a, 2010b), while the crisis in urban governance has fully exposed the rapid undermining of Zimbabwe's bureaucracies through politicisation of state institutions and displacement of technical expertise (McGregor 2013; Dorman 2015).

[49] FGD, Glen Norah, 7 October 2015.

What then does this study of cholera contribute to our growing understanding of urban politics? The cholera outbreak is a unique prism for viewing the interconnections and convergence of the multiple facets of Zimbabwe's urban crisis. The stories told in this chapter explicitly link the cholera outbreak to an array of socio-material processes (particularly the collapse of Zimbabwe's public health infrastructure discussed in Chapter 2), to the failures of urban governance, to the electoral violence of 2008, to economic strategies of survival, and to the arbitrary, spectacular and violent actions of the state. The cholera outbreak allows us to see how these facets of Zimbabwe's crisis converged, mediated and differentiated human life according to such social and economic markers as class, location, political party affiliation, gender and age. This convergence, mediation and differentiation are captured pithily by Samuel Muchero's phrase, 'everything made everything else very difficult'. But this, of course, is especially true of the urban poor of the high-density townships.

For township residents, the outbreak became an important site of evaluating the legitimacy of the ruling government, of venting anger at ZANU(PF)'s manifest failings, and of 'making do' (Jones 2010b) when the state was unable or unwilling to deliver. Cholera instantiated the politics of disposability, the politics of expectation and the politics of adaptation as political subjectivities. Through the cholera stories collated and documented here, my interlocutors, while speaking from an apparent position of victimhood, articulate their expectations of political authority, lay claims to substantive citizenship indexed by access to public services and infrastructural development of the townships, and they discredit what they see as failing bureaucratic institutions. Such claims to substantive citizenship help to explain the ambivalent reception of the salvation agenda, delivered by international humanitarian NGOs. My interlocutors were thankful for the palliation of emergency relief, yet they also insisted that such measures were an inadequate, often inequitable stop-gap unable to attend to the predisposing, precipitating and perpetuating factors that led to the cholera outbreak

Lastly, this chapter has demonstrated the layers of meaning with which an epidemic is endowed even years after its occurrence. Evidently, cholera has been committed to historical memory as an integral component of the nadir of Zimbabwe's political crisis and socio-economic collapse. For many townships residents, much like the doctors and civil servants discussed in preceding chapters, cholera signals the lost *telos* of Zimbabwe's liberation ideals. When Chido and Gamu spoke of living and dying in poverty, they reflected the political and social effects of truncated horizons for youth, a resignation to a hopeless future. Perhaps most tragically of all, there has been little structural transformation of Harare's high-density townships. Patterns of risk and vulnerability, pre-existing social inequalities have barely shifted. People remain terrified of another cholera outbreak. As Favor said morosely, 'I think this time if cholera comes, it's going to wipe us all out.'[50]

[50] Favor 2015 int.

Conclusion

More to Admire Than to Despise?

Stina said a country is a Coca-Cola bottle that can smash on the floor and disappoint you. One day when we were squatting in the bush after eating guavas, Mukoma Charlie found us and said, You are the most unfortunate children this broken bottle has ever seen. When it was still a country you would all be at school doing some serious learning so you would grow up and be somebodies, but here you are, squatting in the bush, guavas ripping your anuses.

—NoViolet Bulawayo, *We Need New Names*, 2013

I have absolutely no doubt in my mind that it's going to happen again. That's what kills me about Africa. We don't learn from yesteryear. Historians will tell you that when history repeats itself, it's a farce.

—Tendai Biti, Interview, Harare, 2015

The Reproach of Cholera

In the past 200 years, the deadly scourge of cholera has ended millions of lives around the world over the course of seven pandemics. Myron Echenberg's (2011) sweeping book, *Africa in a Time of Cholera: A History of Pandemics from 1817 to the Present*, takes Africa as its vantage point for narrating the *longue durée* history of cholera and its relationship to ever-changing currents in politics, geography and public health. The first six cholera pandemics that spanned the period from 1817 to 1947 were truly global events, with the disease endemic in multiple different regions of the world. The seventh pandemic, from 1947 to the present day, has been defined by the emergence of a new biotype of the cholera pathogen and has primarily affected the African continent. Indeed, by 1990, Africa accounted for 90 per cent of cholera cases reported to the WHO (Glass et al. 1991). The Horn of Africa has been especially vulnerable. Almost all the countries in this region host refugees or have internally displaced populations living in overcrowded temporary settlements with poor sanitary conditions. The worst outbreak prior to the one under present study was among Rwandan refugees in relief camps in Goma, Democratic Republic of the Congo, after the 1994 genocide, resulting in 70,000 cases and 12,000 deaths (Heymann and Rodier 1998). For Echenberg (2011: 134–39), it is the breakdown of public health systems, including modern water and sanitation infrastructures, in war-torn countries as the result of systematic attacks on public health resources and healthcare providers that best explains contemporary cholera as a chiefly African occurrence.

The association of cholera with conflict or ecological destruction is strongly justified. Since Echenberg's work was published, several cholera outbreaks have (re-)emerged in different parts of the world for these very reasons. Most notably, in 2010, cholera outbreaks exploded in Haiti after the earthquake and in Pakistan after epic floods. At the time of this writing, cholera plagues South Sudan and Yemen in the context of protracted civil wars. In the contemporary annals of cholera, however, the outbreak in Zimbabwe arguably remains the most alarming given the absence of war or other major, shocking environmental events. Without recourse to an exogenous explanation for cholera, the Zimbabwean experience documented in this book exemplifies what is true of all such epidemics: every phase and aspect of a disastrous outbreak, from origins to resolution, is to a greater or lesser extent a social and political calculus (see Smith 2006). As one of my informants shouted at the end of an interview, 'I think we have talked enough about cholera. But the last thing I can say is that the main factor causing cholera is politically based. It's politically based. It's politically based. It's politically based.'[1]

In the years following the 2008–09 cholera outbreak, the Zimbabwean government has implemented crucial measures to manage recurrences of the disease. In particular, the Ministry of Health has formulated a comprehensive and sophisticated detection and control plan for epidemic disease through use of its Integrated Disease Surveillance and Response protocol (Government of Zimbabwe: Ministry of Health & Child Welfare 2013). However, this strategy is, by its very nature, reactive; it is designed to address outbreaks when they occur, not to prevent them in the first place. The latter remains

[1] Interview, Resident, Glen Norah, 14 August 2015.

difficult for structural reasons. In the last decade, the Ministry of Health has recorded significant gains in responding to and diminishing the case fatality rates of cholera while also noting that environmental factors – specifically poor and inadequate water supplies, recurrent breakdowns in the sewer systems, inadequate sanitation in both urban and rural settings, poor waste management practices, inadequately supervised food preparation processes, and unplanned overcrowded settlements in urban areas – have rendered diarrhoeal disease endemic in Zimbabwe's cities (Government of Zimbabwe: Ministry of Health & Child Welfare 2013; 2016).

The endemicity of diarrhoeal disease, including cholera and typhoid, in urban Zimbabwe has persisted to an important extent because of a protracted water crisis, which, as I have argued repeatedly, is 'politically based'. After the cholera catastrophe, water management in Harare was transferred from ZINWA back to the city council. Despite this, governance of the capital has continued to be a site of intense political struggle, with water management an ongoing focal point of contestation. The dynamics of interparty conflict discussed in Chapters 2 and 5 have persisted long after the cholera outbreak of 2008–09, as a report from the Zimbabwe Coalition on Debt and Development (Zimbabwe Coalition on Debt and Development 2013: 32) on water management during the Government of National Unity has documented:

> Harare is still proving to be the principal site of the intense city-state struggles, where water has been used as a political trump card. It is also speculated that, the City Council has in the bigger picture continued to experience the wrath of the government personified by the Minister of Local Government, Dr. Ignatious Chombo who has taken it upon himself to ensure that the Movement for Democratic Change-Tsvangirai (MDC-T) party was completely incapacitated where water shortages have instrumentally been used by ZANU PF to wrestle control of the city from the MDC-T party.

While this book has been about the politics of Zimbabwe's catastrophic outbreak of cholera in 2008–09, its insights extend far beyond the period and region under examination. In this book, I have used the ten-month period, in which cholera infected over 98,000 people, claimed over 4,000 lives and fulminated throughout Zimbabwe and southern Africa to become the most extensive cholera outbreak in modern African history, as a prism through which to view multiple debates in politics, history and social structures in a new light. I have argued that cholera was produced by, and in turn reproduced, a multiplicity of socio-political crises pertaining to such concerns as the character of the Zimbabwean state, the nature of structural inequalities in Zimbabwean society, the global humanitarian response to epidemics, and ideational formations in everyday life. In this concluding chapter, I synthesise the book's main arguments and discuss the original contributions that this work makes to scholarship.

A 'Man-Made' Disaster

The first question I posed in this book was: *What were the historical and political-economic factors that account for the origins and scale of the cholera outbreak?* I developed my answer in Chapters 1 and 2, in which I argued that Zimbabwe's cholera outbreak was a 'man-made' disaster. Its 'making' was protracted and path-dependent; it was shaped by historical decisions and non-decisions as well as political conflicts; and it was overdetermined by the collapse of Zimbabwe's public health infrastructure and a multifaceted urban crisis. The making of the outbreak lies at the nexus of two overarching phenomena: (1) the enduring and fraught attempts of an authoritarian bureaucratic state to govern urban spaces based on an aesthetic of orderliness and on principles of socio-political control and (2) the social, political and economic upheaval, known as 'the crisis', which emerged from the late 1990s onwards as the ruling party fought to retain political power against the challenge of a new opposition and its own waning popular legitimacy. Below I briefly synthesise my arguments from Chapters 1 and 2 before stating the original contributions that this analysis makes to academe.

The predisposing, or long-term, factors that led to the cholera outbreak can be traced as far back as the late nineteenth century when Salisbury was founded as the administrative and political capital of Southern Rhodesia. The new colonial state rapidly produced, extended and renovated infrastructures – including the city's water reticulation systems that were initially laid down during the 'municipal revolution' – from the late 1800s through much of the early twentieth century. Reflecting the racist and authoritarian character of the Rhodesian state, these infrastructures enabled a series of constitutive, albeit contested, divisions necessary for the establishment of a colonial vision of urban order based on racial segregation in everyday life. For example, the establishment of water systems in the city discriminated, through piping and water delivery mechanisms, between those who were according full membership to the polity and those for whom the promises of citizenship were deferred or denied (see Anand 2017). Additionally, the social differences actualised by urban infrastructures were consolidated by the accreted laws, policies and techniques of colonial governance.

The growth of Salisbury generated a hierarchy of urban space that has persisted to the present. To caricature, this hierarchy exhibits two poles: at one end, the low-density and affluent north-east, and at the other, a densely populated south-west, where the 'native locations' were created to contain and manage Africans in the city (Yoshikuni 2007). Since the colonial period, the 'native locations' (later the high-density townships of Harare's metropolitan area) have suffered from overcrowding; have received public amenities – such as housing, water and sanitation, and healthcare – on an inconsistent and inadequate basis; and have been subjected to periodic, at times violent, state-led 'slum clearances'. The logics of segregationist rule, social control and appeals to orderliness account for the heavy-handed management of the townships by successive governments.

After independence, Harare experienced a 'galloping urbanism' (Musemwa 2012). High-density townships expanded as formal segregation ended and both national and local government sought to improve the delivery of housing stock and supplies of water and sanitation facilities. Such tasks proved more formidable in implementation than in policy, resulting in an ongoing mismatch between supply and need. Moreover, despite gestures toward transforming high-density areas, little changed with respect to the policies that were applied to them. Colonial era by-laws, plans and statutes largely remained in situ (Dorman 2015), indicating the apparent tension between overturning the racial and socio-economic segregation of Rhodesian city planning and maintaining an inherited sense of modernity and orderliness in urban space.

As high-density neighbourhoods expanded with few new suburbs developed, the shortage of housing compelled impoverished urban arrivals to construct 'illegal' shelters in the townships. In response, the government launched a protracted battle against informal housing from the 1980s onwards through forced evictions, arrests, clearances and demolition exercises. The picture began to change in the 1990s because of an unsustainable 'statist' economy, which hampered many government-led social and redistributive programmes. An overvalued currency; arrears to international lenders; shortages of diverse essential goods for commerce and industry; and the failure to adequately reduce pressures on land and achieve restitution in communal areas all contributed to the weakening of the national economy, the delivery of public services and ZANU(PF)'s political legitimacy (Muzondidya 2009; Alexander 2010; Mlambo 2014; Dorman 2016).

The government adopted a controversial economic structural adjustment package to manage the economy at large. The economic reforms of the 1990s led to a deterioration of urban living conditions. Because of unemployment and retrenchment, Harare's townships accommodated increasing numbers of people, within limited space, who had turned to informal trade to stave off livelihood poverty. Worsening public health standards in terms of overcrowded housing and limited access to clean water and sanitation facilities bedevilled the townships. Reactions to visible urban poverty from the government gradually shifted from 'clear-ups' and the forced removal of 'squatters' to gradual tolerance of the informal economy as the 1990s wore on.

Disaffection with economic decline and mismanagement of public finances, corruption scandals in the ruling party and the country's controversial involvement in the war in the Congo were among the most salient factors that led to the formation of ZANU(PF)'s most robust electoral challenger in the form of the MDC. The ruling party readily deployed a chaotic land reform programme, violence, human rights violations, lawlessness and repression of political opposition to oppose its new rival and entrench its political and financial interests. A rapid decline and implosion of the economy ensued, especially from 2000 onwards. At the same time, the ruling party launched an assault on its bureaucratic institutions through an array of legal, coercive and patronage strategies. This assault, demonstrated starkly in the management of municipal services in urban areas, included the displacement of technical experts and individuals affiliated with the MDC in favour of cadres of workers loyal to ZANU(PF). Decades of capital investment and technical know-how were lost.

An exemplar of such changes with central importance to the cholera outbreak was the creation of ZINWA – the Zimbabwe National Water Authority. As I argued in Chapter 2, ZINWA mismanaged and sabotaged the water reticulation systems in Harare and elsewhere. It did so by taking away responsibility for water management from the municipalities, thereby cutting off many MDC-run councils from a crucial aspect of public service delivery. Additionally, ZINWA fired technical staff who had been working in water delivery and replaced them with party loyalists. This allowed the water authority to redirect funds from water bills to the security sector and to the ruling party. Consequently, when Harare was afflicted by severe water shortages, ZINWA had already disposed of the technical, human and financial resources necessary to supply water, to fix waterworks when pipes burst, and to dispose of sewage safely. Thus, a combination of long-term structural factors such as the siting of the water supply system in the same water catchment zone as the sewage system, the poor maintenance of the contemporary water system since it was first established under colonial rule, the misalignment of water provision to population needs, and strategic choices such as the politicisation of ZINWA and the economic crisis, particularly hyperinflation, all contributed to the material collapse of Harare's hydraulic infrastructure.

On top of the collapse of water supply was a collapse of the healthcare delivery system, itself a consequence of Zimbabwe's political-economic meltdown. Lacking staff, stuff, space and systems, the healthcare delivery sector became a crucial factor in the perpetuation of the cholera outbreak. These health system failures were compounded by dramatic changes in livelihoods for much of the population, including and especially those changes caused by Operation *Murambatsvina*. Homelessness, squalor and infrastructural damage in the townships in combination with fuel and currency shortages engendered and augmented widespread, critical food shortages that triggered a sharp rise in acute malnutrition. Acute malnutrition and hunger induced greater susceptibility to cholera in the population, especially among the poor and the vulnerable, and exacerbated its pathological effects in those affected. By 2008–09, the overlapping crises of the collapsed health system, the multi-level failure of the water reticulation system and the political economy of daily life converged to create a 'perfect storm' for a ruinous cholera outbreak.

By elucidating and explaining the socio-material processes underpinning the cholera outbreak I shed new light on Zimbabwe's post-2000 political crisis. Specifically, I have shown how a combination of the transformation of the bureaucratic state combined with the contentious politics of urban governance to result in a public health disaster. The present book can be read alongside other works that have analysed Zimbabwe's political transformations in specific public arenas such as the courts (Verheul 2013), the military (Tendi 2013), the prisons (Alexander 2013), local government (McGregor 2013) and of course the townships (Potts 2006a; Potts 2006b; Fontein 2009; Jones 2010b; Dorman 2015). By using an epidemic as my entry point into such debates and drawing on Rosenberg's notion of 'configuration', I make a novel contribution to the study of Zimbabwean politics by illuminating the devastatingly synergistic interconnections between different aspects of the crisis. This study of the cholera outbreak opens an expansive and illuminating window into state institutions and their practices, and into the sophisticated network of infrastructures that are essential for the administration of everyday life. My analysis has shown how upstream factors – such as the political-economic meltdown and resultant hyperinflation, the manipulation of law for the control of municipal bodies, and the state's 'slum clearances' and demolition exercises in the name of creating urban order – all came to bear on the more proximal drivers of the outbreak such as collapsed healthcare delivery, failed provision of water and sanitation, food insecurity and unregulated informal trade. In much of the Zimbabweanist literature, the cholera outbreak receives only a passing mention as another item on the depressingly long list of tragedies that marked the crisis years. Yet here I argue that the outbreak allows us to see how different aspects of the crisis related to each other and to understand the cascading consequences of state transformation and the breakdown in health infrastructure.

More broadly, I argue that the study of an epidemic as a socio-political phenomenon contributes to the study of politics revealing as it does how state institutions and public infrastructures are causally implicated in an outbreak in the long and short term, how state institutions and infrastructures interact with each other as an outbreak spreads, and how state institutions and infrastructures encounter non-state entities involved in outbreak prevention and response.

One Disease, Many Crises

The second question I posed in this book was: *How did different organisational entities, communities, and individuals act in response to the cholera outbreak?* To tackle this question, I used the concept of multiple ontologies to show how the cholera epidemic took on a variety of different forms, thus engendering a series of high-stakes crises across a range of social and institutional settings. In turn, I argued that the high-stakes crises of cholera gave rise to fraught and contentious politics as different organisational entities, communities and individuals collided with each other in their attempts to command the narrative about cholera and shape the response to it according to their respective ideologies, institutional mandates and political ambitions. The result was a delayed and initially shambolic humanitarian response that was ultimately streamlined and unified by the urgent moral imperative to save lives. However, I also argued that the emergency response to cholera has not addressed the fundamental causes of the outbreak leaving the high-density areas of Harare at ongoing risk of recurrent diarrhoeal disease outbreaks.

The category of emergency is central to the ontological politics of cholera. In part, this stems from a much wider trend in global politics. The twenty-first century has seen the language of 'emergencies' in Africa gain increasing purchase amidst international concerns about security, conflict and the spread of disease; moreover, this language is frequently linked to moral agendas and discourses of human rights (see, for example, Duffield 2007; Verhoeven 2011; Carrier and Klantschnig 2012). The international political framing and response to epidemics as 'emergencies' has been a defining feature of global health in the new millennium (Rushton 2010; McInnes and Lee 2012; Prince and Marsland 2013; de Waal 2014). However, as I have argued through the conceptual framework of 'emergency politics' (Rubenstein 2015), an epidemic can be many different kinds of emergencies to many different constituencies at the same time. Thus, the question of how to act on an epidemic as an emergency is a political one that pits competing interests, priorities, and worldviews against each other.

In Chapter 3, for example, I looked at how the cholera epidemic became a focal point of intense confrontation and political struggle over its meaning and what to do about it. I began by looking at the constituencies for whom cholera was a humanitarian or human rights emergency. MSF pleaded for 'humanitarian space' as a necessary precondition for delivering 'neutral' aid relief to Zimbabweans given the dire state of the country's public health infrastructure. This conception of humanitarian action was itself closely entangled with the notion of human rights, and such language was mobilised by other local and international NGOs seeking to protect vulnerable people from what they saw as the depredations of Mugabe's government. Groups like PHR and the ICG merged human rights concerns with security implications thereby constructing a 'health-security' nexus when they claimed that Zimbabwe's cholera crisis was a threat to both the well-being of local populations and to peace and security regionally and even internationally. The claims that the cholera outbreak posed a security threat to the region only fed the 'siege mentality' of Mugabe's government. ZANU(PF) thus portrayed cholera as a security threat as well but as a threat emanating from neo-colonial predation in which, consistent with the tenets of 'patriotic history', part of the government claimed that cholera was caused by 'the West' and/or that 'the West's' response to the outbreak was part of a subversive regime-change agenda.

The epidemic became a site of struggle as it presented radically different realities to these conflicting institutions. I demonstrated how these oppositional frames stalled humanitarian action on the outbreak. In practice, many of my interlocutors involved with the organisational and practical response dismissed the political debates about security as merely rhetorical and often nonsensical. For example, I posed the question to Steven Maphosa, the director of the Cholera Command and Control Centre, of whether the cholera outbreak was a security risk either to the Zimbabwean state or to the international community:

> I don't know how because a disease outbreak is a disease outbreak and all you need to do is to control the disease. That's the way I see it. How could it be a regional threat? Political? Security? How? Sometimes there is no time or reason to be accusing each other of certain things. We have an outbreak because of poverty, our infrastructure is not working. I don't know how it would be a security threat rather than a health problem ... and something that you need to work on. Not a matter of security or state security.[2]

Maphosa's response was, in many ways, emblematic of the salvation agenda that I discussed in Chapter 4. I argued that the salvation agenda was the moral and technical discourse that allowed the various agencies and actors involved in the medical humanitarian response to set

[2] Stephen Maphosa 2015 int.

aside their multiple, interlocking disputes over the causes of the epidemic and responsibility for its resolution and to focus instead on averting imminent death. Like Ferguson's (1990) anti-politics machine, the salvation agenda presented a complex political and socio-economic reality as a defined problem amenable to technical fixes. However, unlike the anti-politics machine, the salvation agenda did not extend bureaucratic state power. To the contrary, it exposed the enfeeblement of state institutions as well as the limitations of civil servants in exerting authority over foreign NGOs operating in the country, hitherto almost unheard of in Zimbabwe.

The salvation agenda ultimately brought a plethora of organisations together to act on the cholera outbreak as a straightforward public health emergency. In almost every part of the country, cholera treatment centres were set up as teams of healthcare workers channelled patients through different stages of clinical treatment. At the same time, large groups of volunteers did outreach work in surrounding communities to promote safe hygiene practices while also distributing water treatment tablets and, in some cases, drilling boreholes and erecting water tanks in lieu of piped water supplies. Undoubtedly, tens of thousands of people were saved from cholera, and the disease was likely prevented among hundreds of thousands more.

Nevertheless, the resources and energy poured into the salvation agenda were never intended to be more than short-term. The epidemiologist, Renee Loewenson, insisted in our discussion on the absolute necessity of addressing the underlying material conditions that led to cholera as a preventive measure against future outbreaks. As a comparative example, she told me about work that she participated in to eliminate cholera epidemics in Lusaka through addressing the disease's infrastructural drivers:

> The reason I feel quite strongly that it's important to look at those material conditions is because some of those material conditions still exist today in the cities in Zimbabwe. And unless those conditions are dealt with, you can say what you like about the political circumstance, you're going to get the epidemic again. And it was only quite a massive exercise in Lusaka for example to sort of really clean up the waste collection; and to get the population on board with these issues; and to build a trust with the local authorities; and to plan for the rainy season when this is likely to happen; and to look at improving water supplies in the cities and so on. That's when

cholera will move from being an epidemic or endemic problem to not being there. They've eliminated it.

There is no question that you've got to deal with water, sanitation, food markets, all these kinds of things that would be the reason why you would have it. You've got food markets in Harare and there's no toilets, there is no water supply, but people are selling food. Independent of the political situation, you're going to have a risk of cholera in those circumstances. I worry a little bit about the politicisation to the extent of ignoring the material conditions because I think that's allowing the material conditions to persist.[3]

After the outbreak, no serious efforts were undertaken by humanitarian agencies to change health and hydraulic infrastructures, since such fundamental, long-term development work was seen to fall out of the purview of disaster relief. As Abel Gumbo from the Zimbabwean chapter of the Red Cross captured it, 'We look at saving lives and helping people where there is a problem. But the background to what is happening, we don't usually want to hear that.'[4] It may well be too much to expect humanitarian organisations to do more. After all, long-term work that attends to public health infrastructures is typically the responsibility of the state, often in conjunction with development organisations. What I am arguing here, however, is that the prevailing focus on cholera as a public health emergency during the outbreak eclipsed attention to cholera as a long-term crisis of public health infrastructure precipitated by a short-term political-economic crisis. In this way, cholera was not a 'tipping point' in the political life of Zimbabwean society, as the epidemic disaster has left its underlying determinants intact.

The variegated, oppositional and highly political assertions about the cholera outbreak that I have brought to light through this project invite us to think at a more theoretical level about the nature of epidemics. Beyond the present case study, I suggest that there is analytical value in thinking about epidemics in terms of 'multiple ontologies'. Let me make a quick point of comparison about how this line of thinking might have purchase by considering a different epidemic: West Africa's Ebola epidemic in 2013–16 in which Ebola was acted on as a security threat with devastating effect.

[3] Renee Loewenson 2015 int. [4] Abel Gumbo 2015 int.

Melissa Leach (2015) documents how Ebola spread through countries where war and limited post-conflict recovery have left their legacy in dilapidated infrastructure, impoverished capacities and popular discontent. Before the epidemic struck in 2014, Liberia was recovering slowly from two civil wars spanning the 1989–2003 period while Sierra Leone was recovering from a 1991–2002 war that displaced more than 2 million people and killed more than 50,000. War became an early metaphor to describe the spread of Ebola – 'a war with an enemy that we don't see', as a minister in Liberia put it (cited in Leach 2015: 836) – and thus, as the crisis intensified, fears grew that Ebola would likely precipitate further conflict and state failure (Benton 2017).

In September 2014, MSF used the language of security to urge the governments of rich nations to send military medical and biohazard personnel and equipment to respond to the Ebola crisis (Benton 2017). The recommendation was controversial given MSF's traditionally cautious approach to military involvement in humanitarian emergency response. Additionally, the organisation's call delimited the terms for military involvement to exclude such measures as crowd control, quarantine and containment, and instead to focus on clinical care and improved logistics for the diagnosis and management of patients. MSF's strict guidelines for military involvement optimistically suggested that it was possible to deliver military medicine without military might (Benton 2017).

> This framing, along with MSF's call for military biohazard assets, profoundly shaped international intervention in the final months of 2014 and early 2015. In response to MSF's call for medical reinforcements, U.S. President Barack Obama announced his plan to deploy 3,000 troops to combat Ebola in Liberia, giving rise to a range of critiques. Some of the more compelling critiques were presented in visual form. Brazilian political cartoonist Latuff, for example, penned a cartoon captioned 'Obama to send 3,000 troops to fight Ebola in Liberia . . .' In the cartoon, Liberia is a man sick in bed with Ebola. U.S. soldiers in combat gear, guns raised, kick open his bedroom door as they shout, 'Humanitarian aid!' (Benton 2017: 28)

Military personnel in humanitarian situations operate in a nebulous zone between care on one hand and security and coercion on the other. Efforts to demilitarise and downplay the coercive effects of public health require dialogue and deep understanding of local political and social conflicts. More widely, security approaches to public health tend to share similar problems with military approaches to humanitarian assistance. In any outbreak, public health measures entail a degree of coercion as they often require individuals to prioritise community protection. During the Ebola crisis, however, official health security approaches emanating from the West coupled with domestic security concerns resulted in strategies of containment, coercion and criminalisation manifest as state-sponsored violence against 'recalcitrant' communities (those seen as uncooperative with epidemic control procedures) as well as the hyper-vigilance and policing of cross-border mobility. As Paul Farmer (2001a) has argued, such measures are founded on 'an approach which puts physicians and public health personnel in the position of border guards' and undermines the kind of 'solidarity and mutual support' needed to bring an epidemic under control. Additionally, these measures profoundly alienated the very people in need of care, solidarity and support and prolonged the outbreak in the process (Benton 2017).

Recent scholarship on Ebola is highlighting the embeddedness of the disease in complex political (Anderson and Beresford 2016), structural (Leach 2015), historical (Packard 2016) and socio-cultural (Richards 2016) processes. Thinking of the disease according to its multiple ontologies potentially unifies these different strands of analysis. Furthermore, political, policy and public health responses that seek to prevent or mitigate potentially disastrous epidemics must engage with their plurality simultaneously. As I asserted in the Introduction and have argued throughout this book, epidemics are many things at the same time: they are biological phenomena, an infectious disease occurring through a given population in excess of normal expectancy; they are social phenomena, as they spread through populations in socially patterned ways; they are historical phenomena, often the culmination of multi-scalar, political-economic processes that obtain over time; and they are political phenomena, as the declaration of an epidemic is almost always followed by political contests over the attention, resources and priority that said epidemic should receive. They are never only emergencies or only security threats. Such a limited take on epidemics must be challenged through the wider purviews that this book has suggested.

Subjectivity and Crisis

The third, and final, question I posed in this book was: *How has the cholera outbreak been committed to historical memory and what political subjectivities has the epidemic generated?* Throughout this book, I have looked at the myriad meanings, memories and narratives the epidemic has left in its wake across public institutions and in civic life. For the clear majority of my informants, the outbreak aroused public anger and outrage at the government for its causal role in the epidemic and in the inadequacy of its relief efforts. However, this anger has not translated into any effective political mobilisation or permanent change. What I have shown in this work is the sense of both political indignation and impotence that cholera has left in its aftermath. More specifically, I argued that the multiple ontologies of cholera appeared in my informants' narratives as they committed the epidemic to historical memory as a health crisis, a political-economic crisis, and a social crisis as well as a crisis of expectations, history and social identity. As such, the cholera outbreak was intensely generative of subjectivities. In my interviews with township residents, healthcare professionals, activists, journalists and civil servants, I have identified three frequently recurring themes that marked the political subjectivities that emerged during and after the cholera outbreak. These themes were expressed in different ways and to different degrees by my interlocutors. I do not claim that they were universal, but rather that they were ubiquitous. Because of the cholera outbreak, many of my interviewees felt abandoned by the state, and thus they simultaneously expressed anger at and disapproval of its pernicious actions and tremendous failures (a politics of disposability); they articulated a strong normative belief, grounded in historical experience, that the state should be the provider of public goods to citizens on an equitable basis (a politics of expectation); and they adopted diverse survival strategies in response to the cholera outbreak and the wider crisis (a politics of adaptation).

In the high-density township of Glen Norah, I first spoke with Chido and Gamu, two teenage girls who have appeared often in different parts of this book. By their own reckoning, they were born in poverty, live in poverty and will die in poverty.[5] Their political consciousness

[5] Chido 2015 int.

has come into being at the nadir of Zimbabwe's crisis. For them, the cholera outbreak, the political violence, the daily hardship and the implacable sense of loss that defined 2008 etched itself on their minds, leaving them terrified of the depths to which the country could sink. The girls, like other township residents in Harare, are only too aware that the promises of citizenship are only fitfully delivered, even to those who have all the necessary documents that establish their claims to the city (see Anand 2017).

The stories told in Chapter 5 make clear that my interlocutors' everyday experiences of their citizenship entitlements were only tenuously related to their formal status as Zimbabwean citizens or their governmental status as being eligible for water services and healthcare. As such, cholera, like other outbreaks, reveal how substantive citizenship is constituted and indexed by access to public services and violated by anachronistic physical infrastructures, such as the outdated waterworks in their community, or by the arbitrary demolition exercises of the state, such as Operation *Murambatsvina* or indeed more recent upheavals that took place while I was conducting these very interviews:

GAMU: Did you read the news on Wednesday or Thursday about Budiriro houses being destroyed?

FAVOR: Yes, they are destroying homes.

SC: I saw that, they are destroying homes, this has happened many times though.

CHIDO: Whoever made that decision is sitting in the comfort of his home in Borrowdale right now.

CHIDO: Because when they started building those homes, they said it would be better if people had shelter but now they are destroying the shelter. No shelter. Nothing at all. I can't live in this place, it's better abroad.[6]

Outbreaks like cholera always produce and reflect social and political difference. They mark the contours of abandonment, abjection and exclusion. Citizenship is thereby actualised by situated and quotidian encounters with different institutions and officials of the state and political subjectivities are born out of these encounters. An outbreak brings such encounters with the state to vivid light in every phase and aspect of its unfolding from origins to resolution. For my informants in

[6] Group interview with Favor, Chido and Gamu in Glen Norah, 2015.

high-density areas, these encounters led many of them to believe that the state is a sinister institution. Favor, for example, explained to me that, 'People were saying maybe [cholera is] biological warfare, somebody sprayed something in water tanks' as a punishment for 'voting the wrong way'.[7] Others lamented what they saw as malign neglect on the part of the government, repeatedly stating that the ruling party was entirely indifferent to their suffering leaving a humanitarian response to be delivered by foreigners.

At the same time, my interlocutors continued to express expectations that the state can and should deliver public goods – as an elderly man in Budiriro told me: 'In fact, the government should take care of its own people but when people are coming from outside to help that definitely means that there is lack of responsibility proper.'[8] For Tunga, the young doctor in Chapter 4 who volunteered as a medical student to work in cholera treatment centres through Celebration Health, the cholera outbreak triggered a jarring inner turmoil. He expressed horror at the gruesome deaths of cholera that he recognised as being caused by the failed political leadership of a party that he once devotedly followed. Like the character in NoViolet Bulawayo's poignant novel, *We Need New Names*, whom I have quoted in the epigraph to this chapter, Tunga spoke with a sense of longing and loss for the days when Zimbabwe was a 'good, functional country'.[9]

The suffering induced by cholera inspired in Tunga a sense of moral and civic duty to give life-saving treatment to those in need. At the same time, he felt that by standing in where the state had failed he was somehow complicit in supporting an intolerable political situation by mitigating its worst consequences. Didier Fassin (2007a) might describe this dilemma as an *aporia* – contradictions that are both constitutive of the humanitarian project and effectively insurmountable within the existing political order. If we were to shift our attention to Dr Portia Manangazira, in the Ministry of Health, we would see that the imperative of delivering professional services in the midst of a political crisis might be layered with even more complexity than the humanitarian *aporia*. For Max Weber, 'bureaucracy … presupposes an ethical formation on the part of the bureaucrat, a bureaucratic vocation, as opposed to a more or less blind obedience to rules and

[7] Favor 2015 int. [8] Elderly man 2015 int. [9] Tunga 2015 int.

orders' (Osborne 1994: 309). In their professional practice, officials are compelled to act in complex normative universes for which this ideal image of bureaucratic vocation only presents one direction among many others such as partisan loyalty, patron–client relationships or subordination to the security apparatus (Bierschenk 2014). Yet Manangazira is not unique in adhering to a professional ethic of civil service in the thick of Zimbabwe's crisis (see Alexander 2013; Alexander and McGregor 2013; McGregor 2013; Verheul 2013). Accordingly, Alexander (2013: 810) argues:

> The point is not to insist on ideal forms or to measure deviation from them; it is to argue that an important aspect of understanding political change requires asking how formal state institutions are conceived and how they claim and wield authority from the point of view of their actors. This requires a consideration of changes both in civil servants' practice and in the normative and narrative constructions by which the boundaries of (legitimate) state institutions are marked.

For both Tunga and Portia Manangazira, cholera was certainly a medical emergency to which they applied their clinical and public health training, but it was so much more than that. It was a crisis of social identity, as I have just outlined, and it was a political crisis that delineated, with life-and-death consequences, the hierarchies of citizenship in Zimbabwe. Both individuals firmly expressed to me their normative expectations of state–society relations predicated on professional, robust and equitable service delivery for 'ordinary Zimbabweans'; in their view, receipt of public service should not depend on access to patronage or claims to political authority but is a pre-political entitlement.

Lastly, I have discussed how citizens adapted to their sense of abandonment and dispossession by the state and how they negotiated the manifold challenges of the crisis years. The stories told in my focus group discussions with sex workers bear profound testament to this. I was deeply struck by the closing remarks of one of the participants of my focus group in Glen Norah. I quote her briefly again here:

> For us who survived, it taught us perseverance and it also taught us that there is a god. We didn't survive because we are clever or we are intelligent but I think it's by the grace of god that we survived. It brought out a strong Zimbabwean. Form all that experience we became a strong people because

we know that we can survive anything. That year we should have died but because we survived, we now know that we can survive anything.[10]

I was both inspired and troubled by this remark. At first, I understood the statement through the idiom of 'resilience' that has become *de rigueur* in a wave of writing about the pervasiveness of 'neoliberal subjectivities' in humanitarian emergencies. As discussed in the Introduction, emergencies, according to this literature, are presented as an opportunity to manage precariousness and risk. Both humanitarians the state, when they adopt this vision of resilience, aim to help individuals become robust, adaptable, entrepreneurial citizens.

After further reflection, I have concluded that this version of resilience is not the subjectivity being articulated by my interviewees. When considered in tandem with the 'politics of disposability' and the 'politics of expectation' that I have already discussed, then it seems to me that my informants do not imagine their world in post-political terms of self-organisation and survival alone. Adaptation and survival during acute and profound crises might be necessary but they do not dissolve all long-term political expectations in the popular imagination. Crises for my informants have a political basis ('political aetiologies') and a political solution. Disenchantment and frustration with existing political parties, governance structures and individual politicians therefore does not necessarily mean a fundamental or complete abandonment of politics or the state. Even at a time of crisis, the state remains a pre-eminent referent point for collective notions of public welfare, rights and social belonging. Indeed, township residents' publicly articulated rage at the government for its causal role in, and failure to respond to, the cholera outbreak speaks to a much deeper and more widespread aspiration for substantive citizenship based on political rights, social recognition and access to high-quality public services delivered by a robust, responsible state. The success or failure of this aspiration, however, is another matter.

I spoke in the introduction of my interviews as a collaborative alliance between my interlocutors and myself. When conducting my fieldwork, my discussions with those who survived the outbreak were contemplative encounters in which we jointly thought about how and

[10] FGD, Glen Norah, 7 October 2015.

why the cholera outbreak occurred, how it shattered lives and how it was linked to many other problems obtaining in the country. Theoretical notions such as 'multiple ontologies' and 'political subjectivities' were inspired by these conversations and through the stories I was told. Ultimately, the politics of disposability, the politics of expectation and the politics of adaptation are 'mirrors held up to society' (Rosenberg 1992) revealing differences of political ideology, economic power, social experience as well as the distinct terrors that haunt different populations and the particular aspirations they cling to for hope (Briggs and Mantini-Briggs 2004).

Final Reflections

Disastrous epidemics, such as Zimbabwe's cholera outbreak in 2008 and 2009, deserve 'our attention for what they contribute to a general history of society as much as for what they contribute to the history of illness or medicine' (Fassin 2007b: 32). By listening to, reflecting upon and compiling the stories documented in this book and by writing about the awful tragedy that was cholera with affect and connection, I hope that I have provided a new perspective on a dark time in Zimbabwe's recent history. Through this work, I have immersed myself in stories of how people suffer from, treat, manage and argue about a hideous disease. I have also shown how a disease touches virtually every aspect of social and political life, thereby making the dense and intricate linkages between history and political economy, infrastructures and public services, social relations and individual bodies much more apparent.

As I talked with each of my interviewees, I became intensely aware of my detachment from the events of 2008–09. In the Introduction, I described cholera as a visceral experience – one that induces tremendous physical pain, one whose ugly symptoms evoke shame and humiliation, and one that makes plain how vulnerable and resilient bodies can be. Writing about such experiences in a reflective and considered way over a long period of time is a far cry from confronting the immediacy of cholera in the laboratory, in the clinic, in the home or in official buildings where policy decisions are made. Each of my informants spoke with depth and candour, with sharpness of memory, and with expressions of disgust and remorse that cannot be conveyed adequately by words on a page. Indeed, I am not sure how well

I grasped just what it was like to live through such an experience. Perhaps it was simply ineffable.

Nevertheless, the analytical distance afforded to me by such a project comes with its own unique perspective. What I lack in depth of any one experience, I claim back through a more panoramic view of how cholera infiltrated different social, institutional and political settings. This wide-ranging view has impressed upon me that the cholera outbreak was most salient, not for the dramatic character of its particular events, but for its exposition of how terrifying and fatal Zimbabwe's post-2000 political-economic crisis was and of how deep into history the origins of a seemingly short-term emergency can extend. Tendai Biti said to me at the end of our conversation, 'I have absolutely no doubt in my mind that it's going to happen again. That's what kills me about Africa. We don't learn from yesteryear. Historians will tell you that when history repeats itself, it's a farce.'[11] It is my sincere hope that this book presents vital lessons from yesteryear such that we, as Zimbabweans, prevent the tragic farce of another cholera outbreak.

As a final thought, this book has been about suffering and about political failures. But it has also been about hope. When disaster occurs, when political life appears bleak, when deadly illnesses strike with callous disregard, there is always hope to be found in the qualities of compassion, care and creativity shown by people who, far too often, are the unsung heroes of history and in whom the possibility of a more equitable future resides. For these reasons, and to paraphrase Albert Camus (1967) for the last time, what I have learnt in a time of pestilence is that there is much more to admire in humanity than to despise.

[11] Tendai Biti 2015 int.

References

Primary Sources: Interviews and Focus Group Discussions

Informant	Position/Affiliation	Location	Date (2015/16)
Brian Patrick	International Humanitarian Organisation	London	6 July
Nurse	City of Harare Health Services	Mbare	6 August
Favor's Mother-in-law	Resident	Budiriro	10 August
Favor	Resident	Budiriro	10 August
Chido and Gamu	Residents	Glen Norah	14 August
Residents		Glen Norah	14 August
Abel Gumbo	Zimbabwe Red Cross Society	Harare	17 August
Tsitsi	Resident of Kuwadzana	Harare	17 August
Amanda Chikaura	Journalist	Harare	2 September
Samuel Muchero	Teacher at Glen View Primary School	Glen Norah	2 September
Tungamirai Mhuka	Celebration Health	Harare	6 September
Water, Sanitation and Hygiene Specialist 1	Oxfam	Harare	8 September

(*cont.*)

Informant	Position/Affiliation	Location	Date (2015/16)
Water, Sanitation and Hygiene Specialist 2	Oxfam	Harare	8 September
Portia Manangazira	Ministry of Health and Child Welfare	Harare	9 September
Kuda Katurura	Celebration Health	Harare	10 September
David Sanders	Physicians for Human Rights	Johannesburg	12 September
Boniface Nzara	UNICEF	Harare	15 September
Fungai Machiori	Journalist	Harare	15 September
Glanis Changachirere	Activist	Harare	16 September
Goldberg Mangwadu	Ministry of Health and Child Welfare	Harare	16 September
Kumbirai Samuriwo	Journalist	Harare	16 September
Tendai Garwe	Radio personality	Harare	16 September
Aid Worker	International Rescue Committee	Harare	18 September
Stanley Midzi	Ministry of Health and Child Welfare & WHO	Harare	22 September
Audrey	Resident	Hopley Farm	23 September
Chipo	Resident	Hopley Farm	23 September
Focus Group Discussion	Residents	Hopley Farm	23 September
Brian Lunga	Journalist	Harare	24 September
Steven Maphosa	WHO	Harare	24 September
Freeblessing Murahwa	Celebration Health	Harare	25 September
Reuben Akili	Combined Harare Residents Association	Harare	25 September
Elderly couple	Residents	Budiriro	27 September
Young man	Resident	Budiriro	27 September

(*cont.*)

Informant	Position/Affiliation	Location	Date (2015/16)
Kumbirai Mafunda	Zimbabwe Lawyers for Human rights	Harare	1 October
Rue Bonde	Zimbabwe Association of Doctors for Human Rights	Harare	2 October
Margaret Borok	Medical School, University of Zimbabwe	Harare	5 October
Health Activist	Counselling Services Unit	Harare	6 October
Focus Group Discussion	Residents	Dzivarasekwa	7 October
Focus Group Discussion	Residents	Glen Norah	7 October
Ajay Paul	German Agro-Action	Harare	8 October
Health Activist	Zimbabwe Association of Doctors for Human Rights	Harare	8 October
Health Activist	Zimbabwe Association of Doctors for Human Rights	Harare	8 October
Itai Rusike	Community Working Group on Health	Harare	12 October
Henry Madzorera	Former Minister of Health, 2009–2013	Kwekwe	16 October
Nurse	City of Harare Health Services	Harare	21 October
Douglas Gwatidzo	Zimbabwe Association of Doctors for Human Rights	Harare	26 October
Sesel Zvidzai	Former Deputy Minister of Local Government, 2009–2013	Harare	26 October

(*cont.*)

Informant	Position/Affiliation	Location	Date (2015/16)
Civil Society Activist		Harare	27 October
Ish Mafundikwa	Journalist	Harare	28 October
Julie Stewart	Women's Law Centre, University of Zimbabwe	Harare	28 October
Eldred Masunungure	Professor of Political Studies, University of Zimbabwe	Harare	30 October
Maria	Resident of Norton	Harare	31 October
Paida	Resident of Norton	Harare	31 October
Mike Davies	Combined Harare Residents Association	Skype	2 November
Madzudzo Pawadyira	Ministry of Local Government	Harare	11 November
Andrew Reid	Celebration Health	Harare	12 November
Ben Henson	UNICEF Consultant	Harare	12 November
Everjoice Win	Activist, Development Worker	Skype	12 November
Rene Loewenson	Epidemiologist	Harare	14 November
Tendai Biti	Former Minister of Finance, 2009–2013	Harare	16 November
Ben Mbaura	Institute of Migration	Harare	17 November
Aid Worker	Institute of Migration	Harare	17 November
Sikhanyiso Moyo	Kadoma City Council	Kadoma	17 November
Rashida Ferrand	London School of Hygiene and Tropical Medicine	Harare	23 November
Toendepi Kamusuwe	ActionAid	Harare	23 November
Jabu Ngwenya	Celebration Health	Skype	24 November
Resident		Budiriro	25 November
James Munyaradzi	NGO Worker, Resident of Chitungwiza	Harare	18 December
Peter Morris	Civil Engineer	Harare	7 January

Secondary Sources: Bibliography

Abu-Sada, Caroline. 2012. *In the Eyes of Others: How People in Crises Perceive Humanitarian Aid*. New York: MSF-USA.

Alao, Abiodun. 2012. *Mugabe and the Politics of Security*. Montreal: McGill-Queen's University Press.

Alexander, Jocelyn. 2006. *The Unsettled Land: State-Making & the Politics of Land in Zimbabwe, 1893–2003*. Oxford: James Currey.

2010. "Zimbabwe since 1997: Land & the Legacies of War." In *Turning Points in African Democracy*, edited by Abdul Raufu Mustapha and Lindsay Whitfield, 185–201. Suffolk: James Currey.

2013. "Militarisation and State Institutions: 'Professionals' and 'Soldiers' inside the Zimbabwe Prison Service." *Journal of Southern African Studies* 39 (4): 807–28.

Alexander, Jocelyn, and JoAnn McGregor. 2013. "Introduction: Politics, Patronage and Violence in Zimbabwe." *Journal of Southern African Studies* 39 (4): 749–63.

Alexander, Jocelyn, JoAnn McGregor and Terence O. Ranger. 2000. *Violence and Memory: One Hundred Years in the "Dark Forests" of Matabeleland*. Oxford: James Currey.

Alexander, Jocelyn, and Kudakwashe Chitofiri. 2010. "The Consequences of Violent Politics in Norton, Zimbabwe." *The Round Table* 99 (411): 673–86.

Anand, Nikhil. 2017. *Hydraulic City: Water and the Infrastructures of Citizenship in Mumbai*. Durham & London: Duke University Press.

Anderson, Emma-Louise, and Alexander Beresford. 2016. "Infectious Injustice: The Political Foundations of the Ebola Crisis in Sierra Leone." *Third World Quarterly* 37 (3): 468–86.

Arnold, David. 1986. "Cholera and Colonialism in British India." *The Past and Present Society* 113: 118–51.

Auret, Diana. 1990. *A Decade of Development: Zimbabwe 1980–1990*. Harare: Mambo Press.

Awah, Paschal Kum, and Peter Phillimore. 2008. "Diabetes, Medicine and Modernity in Cameroon." *Africa* 78 (4): 475–95.

Bassett, Mary Travis, Leon Bijlmakers and David M. Sanders. 1997. "Professionalism, Patient Satisfaction and Quality of Health Care: Experience during Zimbabwe's Structural Adjustment Programme." *Social Science & Medicine* 45 (12): 1845–52.

Bayart, Jean-Francois. 1986. "Civil Society in Africa." In *Political Domination in Africa: Reflections on the Limits of Power*, edited by Patrick Chabal, 109–25. Cambridge: Cambridge University Press.

2000. "Africa in the World: A History of Extraversion." *African Affairs* 99 (395): 217–67.

BBC. 2008. "UK Caused Cholera, Says Zimbabwe." *BBC News*. http://news.bbc.co.uk/1/hi/world/africa/7780728.stm.

Beach, David. 1999. "Zimbabwe: Pre-colonial History, Demographic Disaster and the University." *Zambezia* 26 (1): 5–33.

Behuria, Pritish, Lars Buur and Hazel Gray. 2017. "Research Note: Studying Political Settlements in Africa." *African Affairs* 116 (464): 508–25.

Benton, Adia. 2017. "Whose Security? Militarization and Securitization During West Africa's Ebola Outbreak." In *The Politics of Fear: Médecins sans Frontières and the West African Ebola Epidemic*, edited by Michiel Hofman and Sokhieng Au, 25–50. Oxford & New York: Oxford University Press.

Beukes, Suzanne Mary. 2013. "Transition Fund Breathes New Life into Zimbabwe's Health System." *UNICEF*. www.unicef.org/infobycountry/zimbabwe_69816.html.

Bierschenk, Thomas. 2014. "Sedimentation, Fragmentation and Normative Double-Blinds in (West) African Public Services." In *States at Work: Dynamics of African Bureaucracies*, edited by Thomas Bierschenk and Jean-Pierre Olivier de Sardan, 221–45. Leiden: Brill Academic Publishers.

Bierschenk, Thomas, and Jean-Pierre Olivier de Sardan. 2014. "Studying the Dynamics of African Bureaucracies: An Introduction to States at Work." In *States At Work: Dynamics of African Bureaucracies*, edited by Thomas Bierschenk and Jean-Pierre Olivier de Sardan, 1–33. Leiden: Brill Academic Publishers.

Bijlmakers, Leon A., Mary T. Bassett and David Sanders. 1996. *Health and Structural Adjustment in Rural and Urban Zimbabwe*. Uppsala: Nordiska Afrikainstitutet.

Blundo, Giorgio, and Jean-Pierre Olivier de Sardan. 2006. *Everyday Corruption and the State: Citizens and Public Officials in Africa*. London: Zed Books.

Blundo, Giorgio, and Pierre-Yves Le Meur. 2009. *The Governance of Daily Life in Africa: Ethnographic Explorations of Public and Collective Services*. Boston: Brill Academic Publishers.

Bolt, Maxim. 2012. "Waged Entrepreneurs, Policed Informality: Work, the Regulation of Space and the Economy of the Zimbabwean-South African Border." *Africa* 82 (1): 111–30.

2015. *Zimbabwe's Migrants and South Africa's Border Farms: The Roots of Impermanence*. New York: Cambridge University Press.

Bond, Patrick. 2007. "Competing Explanations of Zimbabwe's Long Economic Crisis." *Safundi* 8 (2): 149–81.

Bourne, Richard. 2011. *Catastrophe: What Went Wrong in Zimbabwe?* London & New York: Zed Books.

Bratton, Michael. 2014. *Power Politics in Zimbabwe*. Boulder: Lynne Rienner Publishers.

Bratton, Michael, and Nicolas Van De Walle. 1994. "Neopatrimonial Regimes and Political Transitions in Africa." *World Politics* 46 (4): 453–89.

Briggs, Charles L., and Clara Mantini-Briggs. 2004. *Stories in the Time of Cholera Racial Profiling during a Medical Nightmare*. Berkeley: University of California Press.

Buzan, Barry, Ole Wæver and Jaap de Wilde. 1999. *Security: A New Framework for Analysis*. Boulder: Lynne Rienner Publishers.

Calhoun, Craig. 2003. "Afterword: Why Historical Sociology?" In *Handbook of Historical Sociology*, edited by Gerard Delanty and Engin F. Isin, 383–94. London: SAGE Publications.

Cameron, Hazel. 2017. "The Matabeleland Massacres: Britain's Wilful Blindness." *The International History Review*, December. doi:10.1080/07075332.2017.1309561.

Camus, Albert. 1967. *The Plague*. London: Penguin Modern Classics.

Carmody, Pdraig, and Scott Taylor. 2003. "Industry and the Urban Sector in Zimbabwe's Political Economy." *African Studies Quarterly* 7 (2–3): 53–80.

Carpenter, Charles C. J. 1976. "Treatment of Cholera: Tradition and Authority Versus Science, Reason, and Humanity." *Johns Hopkins Medical Journal* 139 (4): 153–62.

Carrier, Neil, and Gernot Klantschnig. 2012. *Africa and the War on Drugs*. London & New York: Zed Books.

Catholic Commission for Justice and Peace in Zimbabwe. 1997. *Breaking the Silence: Building Trust. A Report on the Disturbances in Matabeleland the Midlands, 1980–1988*. Harare: CCJP & LRF.

Chabal, Patrick. 1986. "Introduction: Thinking about Politics in Africa." In *Political Domination in Africa: Reflections on the Limits of Power*, edited by Patrick Chabal, 1–16. Cambridge: Cambridge University Press.

Chabal, Patrick, and Jean-Pascal Daloz. 1999. *Africa Works: Disorder as Political Instrument*. Oxford: James Currey.

Chhotray, Vasudha. 2014. "Disaster Relief and the Indian State: Lessons for Just Citizenship." *Geoforum* 54: 217–25.

Chikanda, Abel. 2005. *Medical Leave: The Exodus of Health Professionals from Zimbabwe*. Cape Town: Idasa.

Chimhowu, Amos, and Daniel S Tevera. 1998. "Urban Growth, Poverty and Backyard Shanties in Harare, Zimbabwe." *Geographical Journal of Zimbabwe* 29: 11–22.

Chiumbu, Sarah, and Muchaparara Musemwa. 2012. *Crisis! What Crisis?: The Multiple Dimensions of the Zimbabwean Crisis*. Cape Town: HSRC Press.

Choi, Vivian. 2013. "Disaster: Translation." *Cultural Anthropology Website*. https://culanth.org/fieldsights/150-disaster-translation.

Clapham, Christopher. 2017. *The Horn of Africa: State Formation and Decay*. London: Hurst and Company.

Cohen, Stanley. 2001. *States of Denial: Knowing about Atrocities and Suffering*. Cambridge: Polity Press.

Comaroff, Jean. 2007. "Beyond Bare Life: AIDS, (Bio)Politics, and the Neoliberal Order." *Public Culture* 19 (1): 197–219.

Cook, Richard I. 1998. *How Complex Systems Fail*. Chicago: University of Chicago, Cognitive Technologies Laboratory.

Cooper, Frederick. 2002. *Africa since 1940: The Past of the Present*. Cambridge: Cambridge University Press.

Coutinho, Boniface. 2010. "Sources of Local Government Financing." In *Local Government Reform in Zimbabwe: A Policy Dialogue*, edited by Jaap de Visser, Nico Steytler, and Naison Machingauta, 71–89. Bellville: Community Law Centre.

Cumming, Sioux. 1993. "Post-Colonial Urban Residential Change in Harare: A Case Study." In *Harare: The Growth and Problems of the City*, edited by Zinyama Lovemore, Tevera Daniel, and Cumming Sioux, 153–75. Harare: University of Zimbabwe.

Das, Veena, and Deborah Poole. 2004. *Anthropology in the Margins of the State*. Santa Fe: School of American Research Press.

Davies, D. Hywel. 1986. "Harare, Zimbabwe: Origins, Development and Post-colonial Change." *African Urban Quarterly* 1 (2): 131–38.

de Waal, Alex. 1989. *Famine That Kills: Darfur, Sudan*. Oxford: Oxford University Press.

1997. *Famine Crimes: Politics and the Disaster Relief Industry in Africa*. Oxford: Oxford University Press.

2006. *AIDS and Power: Why There Is No Political Crisis -Yet*. London & New York: Zed Books.

2014. "Militarized Global Health." *Boston Review*, November. www.bostonreview.net/world/alex-de-waal-militarizing-global-health-ebola.

Dieleman, Marjolein, Mark Watson and Chenjerai Sisimayi. 2012. "Impact Assessment of the Zimbabwe Health Worker Retention Scheme. Final Report."

Dorman, Sara Rich. 2015. "'We Have Not Made Anybody Homeless': Regulation and Control of Urban Life in Zimbabwe." *Citizenship Studies* 20 (1): 84–98.

2016. *Understanding Zimbabwe: From Liberation to Authoritarianism*. London: Hurst and Company.

Duffield, Mark. 2007. *Development, Security and Unending War: Governing the World of Peoples*. Cambridge: Polity Press.

2011. "Environmental Terror: Uncertainty, Resilience and the Bunker." *Environmental School of Sociology, Politics and International Studies University of Bristol Working Paper*. www.bristol.ac.uk/spais/research/workingpapers/wpspaisfiles/duffield-0611.pdf.

Dugger, Celia W. 2008. "Cholera Epidemic Sweeping across Crumbling Zimbabwe." *The New York Times*, December 11.

Dzirutwe, MacDonald. 2008. "Mugabe Says Zimbabwe Cholera Outbreak Stopped." *Reuters*, December 11. http://reliefweb.int/report/south-africa/mugabe-says-zimbabwe-cholera-outbreak-stopped.

Echenberg, Myron. 2011. *Africa in the Time of Cholera: A History of Pandemics from 1817 to the Present*. Cambridge: Cambridge University Press.

Edelstein, Michael, David Heymann and Khalid Koser. 2014. "Health Crises and Migration." In *Humanitarian Crises and Migration: Causes, Consequences and Responses*, edited by Susan F. Martin, Sanjula Weerasinghe, and Abbie Taylor, 97–112. London: Routledge.

Englebert, Pierre, and Denis M Tull. 2008. "Postconflict Reconstruction in Africa Flawed Ideas about Failed States." *International Security* 32 (4): 106–39.

Evans, Richard J. 2006. *Death in Hamburg: Society and Politics in the Cholera Years, 1830–1910*. New York: Penguin USA.

Farmer, Paul. 2001a. *Infections and Inequalities: The Modern Plagues*. Berkeley and Los Angeles: University of California Press.

Farmer2001b. "Russia's Tuberculosis Catastrophe." *Project Syndicate*. www.project-syndicate.org/commentary/russia-s-tuberculosis-catas trophe?barrier=accessreg.

Farmer, Paul, Arthur Kleinman, Jim Kim and Matthew Basilico. 2013. *Reimagining Global Health: An Introduction*. Berkeley and Los Angeles: University of California Press.

Fassin, Didier. 2007a. "Humanitarianism as a Politics of Life." *Public Culture* 19 (3): 499–520.

2007b. *When Bodies Remember: Experiences and Politics of AIDS in South Africa*. Berkley and Los Angeles: University of California Press.

Ferguson, James. 1990. *The Anti-Politics Machine: "Development," Depoliticization, and Bureaucratic Power in Lesotho*. Cambridge: Cambridge University Press.

Ferguson, James, and Akhil Gupta. 2002. "Spatializing States: Toward an Ethnography of Neoliberal Governmentality." *American Ethnologist* 29 (4): 981–1002.

Fontein, Joost. 2008. "The Power of Water: Landscape, Water and the State in Southern and Eastern Africa: An Introduction." *Journal of Southern African Studies* 34 (4): 737–56.

2009. "Anticipating the Tsunami: Rumours, Planning and the Arbitrary State in Zimbabwe." *Africa: Journal of the International African Institute* 79 (3): 369–98.

Forsyth, Timothy. 2004. *Critical Political Ecology: The Politics of Environmental Science*. London: Routledge.

Fournier, Christophe, and Jonathan Whittall. 2009. "When the Affected State Causes the Crisis: The Case of Zimbabwe." *Humanitarian Exchange*. www.odihpn.org/humanitarian-exchange-magazine/issue-44.

Gann, L. H., and Peter Duignan. 1970. "Changing Patterns of a White Elite." In *Colonialism in Africa, 1870–1960, The History and Politics of Colonialism 1870–1914, Vol. II*, edited by L. H. Gann and Peter Duignan, 138–39. Cambridge: Cambridge University Press.

Geschiere, Peter. 1988. "Sorcery and the State: Popular Modes of Action among the Maka of Southeast Cameroon." *Critique of Anthropology* 8 (1): 35–63.

Gibbon, Peter. 1995. "Introduction: Structural Adjustment and the Working Poor in Zimbabwe." In *Structural Adjustment and the Working Poor in Zimbabwe: Studies on Labour, Women Informal Sector Workers and Health*, edited by Peter Gibbon, 7–37. Uppsala: Nordiska Afrikainstitutet.

Giroux, Henry A. 2006. "Reading Hurricane Katrina: Race, Class, and the Biopolitics of Disposability." *College Literature* 33 (3): 171–96.

Glaser, Barney, and Anselm Strauss. 1967. *The Discovery of Grounded Research: Strategies for Qualitative Research*. Piscataway: Aldine Transaction.

Glass, Roger. I., Mariam Claeson, Paul A. Blake, Ronald J. Waldman and Nathaniel F. Pierce. 1991. "Cholera in Africa: Lessons on Transmission and Control for Latin America." *The Lancet* 338 (8770): 791–95.

Government of Zimbabwe: Ministry of Health & Child Welfare. 2013. "The National Health Strategy for Zimbabwe, 2009–2013: Equity and Quality in Health: A People's Right." Harare.

2016. "The National Health Strategy for Zimbabwe 2016–2020: Equity and Quality in Health: Leaving No One Behind." www.unicef.org/zimbabwe/National_Health_Strategy_for_Zimbabwe_2016-2020_FINAL.pdf.

Gowans, Stephen. 2008. "Cholera: West's Latest Weapon on Zimbabwe." *The Herald*, December 20.

Guggenheim, Michael. 2014. "Introduction: Disaster as Politics – Politics as Disasters." *The Sociological Review* 16 (S1): 1–16.

Hagmann, Tobias, and Didier Péclard. 2010. "Negotiating Statehood: Dynamics of Power and Domination in Africa." *Development and Change* 41 (4): 539–62.

Hamdy, Sherine F. 2008. "When the State and Your Kidneys Fail: Political Etiologies in an Egyptian Dialysis Ward." *American Ethnologist* 35 (4): 553–69.

Hammar, Amanda, Brian Raftopoulos and Stig Jensen. 2003. *Zimbabwe's Unfinished Business: Rethinking Land, State and Nation in the Context of Crisis*. Harare: Weaver Press.

Hanke, Steve H, and Alex K. F. Kwok. 2009. "On the Measurement of Zimbabwe's Hyperinflation." *Cato Journal* 29 (2): 353–64.

Hansen, Thomas, and Finn Stepputat. 2001. *States of Imagination: Ethnographic Explorations of the Postcolonial State*. Durham: Duke University Press.

Herbst, Jeffrey. 2000. *States and Power in Africa: Comparative Lessons in Authority and Control*. Princeton: Princeton University Press.

Herring, Ann, and Alan C. Swedlund. 2010. "Plagues and Epidemics in Anthropological Perspective." In *Plagues and Epidemics: Infected Spaces Past and Present*, edited by Ann Herring and Alan C. Swedlund, 1–20. London: Bloomsbury Academic.

Heymann, David L., and Guénaël R. Rodier. 1998. "Global Surveillance of Communicable Diseases." *Emerging Infectious Diseases* 4 (3): 362–65.

Hoekman, Thys. 2013. "Testing Ties: Opposition and Power-Sharing Negotiations in Zimbabwe." *Journal of Southern African Studies* 39 (4): 903–20.

Hogan, Barbara. 2008. "Statement by Minister of Health Barbara Hogan on the Outbreak of Cholera in Zimbabwe and South Africa." *ReliefWeb*. https://reliefweb.int/report/south-africa/statement-minister-health-barbara-hogan-outbreak-cholera-zimbabwe-and-south.

Holston, James. 2008. *Insurgent Citizenship: Disjunctions of Democracy and Modernity in Brazil*. Princeton: Princeton University Press.

Hopkins, Antony G. 2000. "Quasi-States, Weak States and the Partition of Africa." *Review of International Studies* 26 (2): 311–20.

Hove-Musekwa, Senelani D., Farai Nyabadza, Christinah Chiyaka, Prasenjit Das, Agraj Tripathi and Zindoga Mukandavire. 2011. "Modelling and Analysis of the Effects of Malnutrition in the Spread of Cholera." *Mathematical and Computer Modelling* 53 (9–10): 1583–95.

Hungwe, Brian. 2008. "The Death Throes of Harare's Hospitals." *BBC News*, November 7. http://news.bbc.co.uk/1/hi/world/africa/7714892.stm.

International Crisis Group. 2008. "Ending Zimbabwe's Nightmare: A Possible Way Forward." Pretoria/Brussels.

IRIN. 2008a. "Cholera Timelime." *Integrated Regional Information Networks*. www.irinnews.org/news/2008/12/05/cholera-timeline.

2008b. "Disaster Unit Deployed in Response to Cholera Outbreak." *Integrated Regional Information Networks*. Harare. November 5. www.irinnews.org/report/81314/zimbabwe-disaster-unit-deployed-in-response-to-cholera-outbreak.

Jackson, Michael. 2002. *The Politics of Storytelling: Violence, Transgression and Intersubjectivity*. Copenhagen: Museum Tusculanum Press.

Jackson, Robert H., and Carl G. Rosberg. 1982. "Why Africa's Weak States Persist: The Empirical and the Juridical in Statehood." *World Politics* 35 (1): 1–24.

Janes, Craig R., and Kitty K. Corbett. 2009. "Anthropology and Global Health." *Annual Review of Anthropology* 38 (1): 167–83.

Jasanoff, Sheila. 2004. "The Idiom of Co-Production." In *States of Knowledge: The Co-Production of Science and the Social Order*, edited by Sheila Jasanoff, 1–12. London: Routledge.

Jones, Jeremy L. 2010a. "Freeze! Movement, Narrative and the Disciplining of Price in Hyperinflationary Zimbabwe." *Social Dynamics* 36 (2): 338–51.

2010b. "'Nothing Is Straight in Zimbabwe': The Rise of the Kukiya-Kiya Economy 2000–2008." *Journal of Southern African Studies* 36 (2): 285–99.

Jones, Will, Ricardo Soares de Oliveira, and Harry Verhoeven. 2013. "Africa's Illiberal State-Builders." *University of Oxford: Refugee Studies Centre*, no. 89. Oxford.

Kamete, Amin. 2006. "The Return of the Jettisoned: ZANU-PF's Crack at 'Re-Urbanising' in Harare." *Journal of Southern African Studies* 32 (2): 255–71.

Karekwaivanene, George. 2012. *Legal Encounters: Law, State and Society in Zimbabwe, c. 1950–1990*. Oxford: Unpublished DPhil Thesis, University of Oxford.

Keen, David. 1991. *The Benefits of Famine: A Political Economy of Famine and Relief in Southwestern Sudan, 1983–1989*. Princeton: Princeton University Press.

Khan, Mushtaq. 1995. "State Failure in Weak States: A Critique of New Institutionalist Explanations." In *New Institutional Economics and Third World Development*, edited by John Harriss, Janet Hunter, and Colin Lewis, 71–86. London: Routledge.

Kleinman, Arthur. 2010. "Four Social Theories for Global Health." *The Lancet* 375 (9725): 1518–19.

Krause, Kristine, and Katharina Schramm. 2011. "Thinking through Political Subjectivity." *African Diaspora* 4: 115–34.

Last, John M. 2001. *A Dictionary of Epidemiology*. New York: Oxford University Press.

Leach, Melissa. 2015. "The Ebola Crisis and Post-2015 Development." *Journal of International Development* 834: 816–34.

Lee, Kelley. 2001. "The Global Dimensions of Cholera." *Global Change and Human Health* 2 (1): 6–17.

Lopman, Ben A., Ruanne Barnabas, Timothy B. Hallett, Constance Nyamukapa, Costa Mundandi, Phyllis Mushati, Geoff P. Garnett and Simon Gregson. 2006. "Assessing Adult Mortality in HIV-1-Afflicted Zimbabwe (1998–2003)." *Bulletin of the World Health Organization* 84 (5): 189–97.

Luque Fernández, Miguel Ángel, Peter R. Mason, Henry Gray, Ariane Bauernfeind, Jean François Fesselet and Peter Maes. 2011. "Descriptive Spatial Analysis of the Cholera Epidemic 2008–2009 in Harare, Zimbabwe: A Secondary Data Analysis." *Transactions of the Royal Society of Tropical Medicine and Hygiene* 105: 38–45.

Luque Fernandez, Miguel A., Michael Schomaker, Peter R Mason, Jean F Fesselet, Yves Baudot, Andrew Boulle and Peter Maes. 2012. "Elevation and Cholera: An Epidemiological Spatial Analysis of the Cholera Epidemic in Harare, Zimbabwe, 2008–2009." *BMC Public Health* 12: 442.

Martinez, Ian. 2002. "The History of the Use of Bacteriological and Chemical Agents during Zimbabwe's Liberation War of 1965–80 by Rhodesian Forces." *Third World Quarterly* 23 (6): 1159–79.

Mason, Peter R. 2009. "Zimbabwe Experiences the Worst Epidemic of Cholera in Africa." *Journal of Infection in Developing Countries* 3 (2): 148–51.

Mbembe, Achille, and Janet Roitman. 1995. "Figures of the Subject in Times of Crisis." *Public Culture* 7 (2): 323–52.

McCulloch, Jock. 2000. *Black Peril, White Virtue: Sexual Crime in Southern Rhodesia, 1902–1935*. Bloomington: Indiana University Press.

McGregor, JoAnn. 2013. "Surveillance and the City: Patronage, Power-Sharing and the Politics of Urban Control in Zimbabwe." *Journal of Southern African Studies* 39 (4): 783–805.

McGregor, JoAnn, and Terence O. Ranger. 2000. "Displacement and Disease: Epidemic and Ideas about Malaria in Matabeleland, Zimbabwe, 1945–1966." *Past & Present* 167: 203–37.

McInnes, Colin, and Kelley Lee. 2012. *Global Health and International Relations*. Cambridge: Polity Press.

Médecins Sans Frontières. 2009a. "Beyond Cholera: Zimbabwe's Worsening Crisis." *International Website of Médecins Sans Frontières (MSF)*. www.msf.org/beyond-cholera-zimbabwes-worsening-crisis.

2009b. "Cholera: 'This Is a Human Being and Should Not Be Treated This Way.'" *International Website of Médecins Sans Frontières (MSF)*. www.msf.org/article/cholera-human-being-and-should-not-be-treated-way.

2009c. "Cholera Has 'Burnt Its Way through' Zimbabwe Villages." *International Website of Médecins Sans Frontières (MSF)*. www.msf.org/en/article/cholera-has-burnt-its-way-through-zimbabwe-villages.

2009d. "No Refuge, Access Denied: Medical and Humanitarian Needs of Zimbabweans in South Africa," www.doctorswithoutborders.org/what-we-do/news-stories/research/no-refuge-access-denied-medical-and-humanitarian-needs-zimbabweans.

2009e. "Press Teleconference on Zimbabwe." www.doctorswithoutborders.org/news-stories/transcript/press-teleconference-zimbabwe#christophe1.

2009f. "The Colour of Cholera." *International Website of Médecins Sans Frontières (MSF)*. www.msf.org/article/colour-cholera.

2009g. "The Force of Argument." *International Website of Médecins Sans Frontières (MSF)*. http://blogs.msf.org/en/staff/blogs/cholera-cholera/the-force-of-argument.

Migdal, Joel S. 1988. *Strong Societies and Weak States: State-Society Relations and State Capabilities in the Third World*. Princeton: Princeton University Press.

Mlambo, Alois S. 2014. *A History of Zimbabwe*. Cambridge: Cambridge University Press.

Mol, Annemarie. 1999. "Ontological Politics. A Word and Some Questions." *The Sociological Review* 47 (1_suppl): 74–89.

2002. *The Body Multiple: Ontology in Medical Practice*. Durham & London: Duke University Press.

Moore, David B, and Brian Raftopoulos. 2012. "Zimbabwe's Democracy of Diminished Expectations." In *Crisis! What Crisis?: The Multiple Dimensions of the Zimbabwean Crisis*, edited by Sarah Chiumbu and Muchaparara Musemwa, 241–67. Cape Town: HSRC Press.

Moyo, Sam, and Paris Yeros. 2007a. "The Radicalised State: Zimbabwe's Interrupted Revolution." *Review of African Political Economy* 34 (111): 103–21.

2007b. "The Zimbabwe Question and the Two Lefts." *Historical Materialism* 15 (3): 171–204.

Muchichwa, Nyasha. 2016. "Working without Pay: Wage Theft in Zimbabwe." International Website of the Solidarity Center. www.solidaritycenter.org/wp-content/uploads/2016/07/Zimbabwe.Working-without-Pay-Wage-Theft-in-Zimbabwe.7.16.pdf.

Mukandavire, Zindoga, Shu Liao, Jin Wang, Holly Gaff, David L Smith, and J Glenn Morris. 2011. "Estimating the Reproductive Numbers for the 2008–2009 Cholera Outbreaks in Zimbabwe." *Proceedings of the National Academy of Sciences of the United States of America* 108 (21): 8767–72.

Musemwa, Muchaparara. 2006. "Disciplining a 'Dissident' City: Hydropolitics in the City of Bulawayo, Matabeleland, Zimbabwe, 1980-1994." *Journal of Southern African Studies* 32 (2): 239–54.

2008a. "Early Struggles over Water: From Private to Public Water Utility in the City of Bulawayo, Zimbabwe, 1894–1924." *Journal of Southern African Studies* 34 (4): 881–98.

2008b. "The Politics of Water in Post-Colonial Zimbabwe, 1980–2007." *African Studies Centre, University of Leiden*, June.

2010. "From 'Sunshine City' to a Landscape of Disaster: The Politics of Water, Sanitation and Disease in Harare, Zimbabwe, 1980–2009." *Journal of Developing Societies* 26 (2): 165–206.

2012. "Perpetuating Colonial Legacies: The Post-Colonial State, Water Crises and the Outbreak of Disease in Harare, Zimbabwe, 1980–2009." In *Crisis! What Crisis?: The Multiple Dimensions of the Zimbabwean Crisis*, edited by Sarah Chiumbu and Muchaparara Musemwa, 3–41. Cape Town: HSRC Press.

Musoni, Francis. 2010. "Operation Murambatsvina and the Politics of Street Vendors in Zimbabwe." *Journal of Southern African Studies* 36 (2): 301–17.

Muzondidya, James. 2009. "From Buoyancy to Crisis, 1980–1997." In *Becoming Zimbabwe: A History from the Pre-Colonial Period to 2008*, edited by Brian Raftopoulos and Alois Mlambo, 167–200. Harare: Weaver Press.

Ndlovu, Thabisani. 2012. "Escaping Home: The Case of Ethnicity and Formal Education in the Migration of Zimbabweans during the Zimbabwean 'Crisis.'" In *Crisis! What Crisis?: The Multiple Dimensions of the Zimbabwean Crisis*, edited by Sarah Chiumbu and Muchaparara Musemwa, 100–121. Cape Town: HSRC Press.

Ndlovu-Gatsheni, Sabelo J. 2009a. "Making Sense of Mugabeism in Local and Global Politics: 'So Blair, Keep Your England and Let Me Keep My Zimbabwe.'" *Third World Quarterly* 30 (6): 1139–58.

2009b. "Mapping Cultural and Colonial Encounters, 1880s–1930s." In *Becoming Zimbabwe: A History from the Pre-colonial Period to 2008*, edited by Brian Raftopoulos and Alois Mlambo, 39–74. Harare: Weaver Press.

Neseni, Noma, and Edward Guzha. 2009. *Evaluation of the WASH Response to the 2008–2009 Zimbabwe Cholera Epidemic and*

Preparedness Planning for Future Outbreaks. Harare: Institute of Water and Sanitation Development.

News24. 2016. "Under Whites, Zim Wasn't Dirty, Minister Says As Cholera Hits Harare." *Special Reports: Zimbabwe*. www.news24.com/Africa/Zimbabwe/under-whites-zim-wasnt-dirty-minister-says-as-cholera-hits-harare-20161022.

Nugent, Paul. 2010. "States and Social Contracts in Africa." *New Left Review* 63 (May–June): 35–68.

Nustad, Knut G. 2001. "Development: The Devil We Know?" *Third World Quarterly* 22 (4): 479–89.

Nuttall, S. 1998. "Telling 'Free' Stories? Memory and Democracy in South African Autobiography since 1994." In *Negotiating the Past: The Making of Memory in South Africa*, edited by Sarah Nuttall and Carli Coetzee, 75–88. Oxford: Oxford University Press.

Ong, Aihwa. 1996. "Cultural Citizenship as Subject-Making: Immigrants Negotiate Racial and Cultural Boundaries in the United States." *Current Anthropology* 37 (5): 737–62.

Osborne, Thomas. 1994. "Bureaucracy as a Vocation: Governmentality and Administration in Nineteenth-century Britain." *Journal of Historical Sociology* 7 (3): 289–313.

Packard, Randall M. 2016. *A History of Global Health: Interventions into the Lives of Other Peoples*. Baltimore, MD: Johns Hopkins University Press.

Patel, Diana. 1984. "Housing the Urban Poor in the Socialist Transformation of Zimbabwe." In *The Political Economy of Zimbabwe*, edited by Michael G. Schatzberg, 182–96. New York City: Praeger.

Patrick, Stewart. 2011. *Weak Links: Fragile States, Global Threats, and International Security*. New York: Oxford University Press.

Pelling, Mark, and Kathleen Dill. 2010. "Disaster Politics: Tipping Points for Change in the Adaptation of Sociopolitical Regimes." *Progress in Human Geography* 34 (1): 21–37.

Phiminister, Ian. 1988. *An Economic and Social History of Zimbabwe, 1890-1948: Capital Accumulation and Class Struggle*. London: Longman Higher Education.

Phimister, Ian, and Brian Raftopoulos. 2004. "Mugabe, Mbeki & the Politics of Anti-Imperialism." *Review of African Political Economy* 31 (101): 385–400.

Physicians for Human Rights 2011. "About PHR." http://physiciansforhumanrights.org/about/.

Potts, Deborah. 2006a. "City Life in Zimbabwe at a Time of Fear and Loathing: Urban Planning, Urban Poverty, and Operation

Murambatsvina." In *Cities in Contemporary Africa*, edited by Martin J. Murray and Garth A. Myers, 265–88. New York: Palgrave Macmillan.

2006b. "'Restoring Order'? Operation Murambatsvina and the Urban Crisis in Zimbabwe." *Journal of Southern African Studies* 32 (2): 273–91.

Potts, Deborah, and C. C. Mutambirwa. 1991. "High-Density Housing in Harare: Commodification and Overcrowding." *Third World Planning Review* 13 (1): 1–25.

Prince, Ruth Jane, and Rebecca Marsland. 2013. *Making and Unmaking Public Health in Africa: Ethnographic and Historical Perspectives*. Athens: Ohio University Press.

Raftopoulos, Brian. 2009. "The Crisis in Zimbabwe, 1998–2008." In *Becoming Zimbabwe: A History from the Pre-colonial Period to 2008*, edited by Brian Raftopoulos and Alois Mlambo, 201–32. Harare: Weaver Press.

Raftopoulos, Brian, and Tsuneo Yoshikuni. 1999. "Introduction." In *Sites of Struggle: Essays in Zimbabwe's Urban History*, edited by Brian Raftopoulos and Tsuneo Yoshikuni, 1–18. Harare: Weaver Press.

Ranger, Terence O. 2004. "Nationalist Historiography, Patriotic History and the History of the Nation: The Struggle over the Past in Zimbabwe." *Journal of Southern African Studies* 30 (2): 215–34.

2007. "City Versus State in Zimbabwe: Colonial Antecedents of the Current Crisis." *Journal of Eastern African Studies* 1 (2): 161–92.

Ranger, Terence O., and Paul Slack. 1995. *Epidemics and Ideas: Essays on the Historical Perception of Pestilence*. Cambridge: Cambridge University Press.

Rao, Rahul. 2013. "Postcolonial Cosmopolitanism: Making Place for Nationalism." In *The Democratic Predicament: Cultural Diversity in Europe and India*, edited by Jyotirmaya Tripathy and Sudarsan Padmanabhan, 165–87. New Delhi: Routledge.

Redfield, Peter. 2005. "Doctors, Borders, and Life in Crisis." *Cultural Anthropology* 20 (3): 328–61.

2011. "The Impossible Problem of Neutrality." In *Forces of Compassion: Humanitarianism Between Ethics and Politics*, edited by Erica Bornstein and Peter Redfield, 53–70. Santa Fe: School for Advanced Research Advanced Press.

Redfield, Peter, and Erica Bornstein. 2011. "An Introduction to the Anthropology of Humanitarianism." In *Forces of Compassion: Humanitarianism between Ethics and Politics*. Santa Fe: School for Advanced Research Advanced Press.

Reno, William. 1999. *Warlord Politics and African States*. Boulder: Lynne Rienner Publishers.

Reserve Bank of Zimbabwe. 2008. "Inflation Rates." www.rbz.co.zw/about/inflation.asp.

Richards, Paul. 2016. *Ebola: How a People's Science Helped End an Epidemic*. London: Zed Books.

Rosen, Armin. 2013. "How the UN Covered Up a Cholera Epidemic in Zimbabwe." *The Atlantic*. www.theatlantic.com/international/archive/2013/04/how-the-un-covered-up-a-cholera-epidemic-in-zimbabwe/274627/.

Rosenberg, Charles E. 1989. "What Is an Epidemic? AIDS in Historical Perspective." *Daedalus* 118 (2): 1–17.

1992. *Explaining Epidemics and Other Studies in the History of Medicine*. Cambridge: Cambridge University Press.

Rotberg, Robert I. 2002. "The New Nature of Nation-State Failure." *The Washington Quarterly* 25 (3): 83–96.

Rubenstein, Jennifer C. 2015. "Emergency Claims and Democratic Action." *Social Philosophy and Policy* 32 (1): 101–26.

Rushton, Simon. 2010. "Framing AIDS: Securitization, Development-ization, Rights-ization." *Global Health Governance* 4 (1): 1–17.

Sapire, Hilary, and Jo Beall. 1995. "Introduction: Urban Change and Urban Studies in Southern Africa." *Journal of Southern African Studies* 21 (1): 3–17.

Scheper-Hughes, Nancy. 1992. *Death without Weeping: The Violence of Everyday Life in Brazil*. Berkeley: University of California Press.

Schoffeleers, Matthew. 1999. "The AIDS Pandemic, the Prophet Billy Chisupe, and the Democratization Process in Malawi." *Journal of Religion in Africa* 29 (4): 406–41.

Scott, James C. 1985. *Weapons of the Weak: Everyday Forms of Peasant Resistance*. New Haven: Yale University Press.

Scott-Smith, Tom. 2014. *Defining Hunger, Redefining Food: Humanitarianism in the Twentieth Century*. Oxford: Unpublished DPhil Thesis, University of Oxford.

2015. "The Fetishism of Humanitarian Objects and the Management of Malnutrition in Emergencies." *Third World Quarterly* 34 (5): 913–28.

2018. "Paradoxes of Resilience: A Review of the World Disasters Report 2016." *Development and Change* 0 (0): 1–16.

Seirlis, Julia Katherine. 2004. "Islands and Autochthons: Coloureds, Space and Belonging in Rhodesia and Zimbabwe." *Journal of Social Archaeology* 4 (3): 405–27.

Sharma, Aradhana, and Akhil Gupta. 2006. *The Anthropology of the State: A Reader*. Malden: Blackwell Publishing.

Sibanda, Nkululeko, and Wongai Zhangazha. 2008. "NGO Ban Worsens Plight Of The Poor." *Zimbabwe Independent*, June 13. www.theindependent.co.zw/2008/06/13/ngo-ban-worsens-plight-of-the-poor/.

Singer, Merrill, and Scott Clair. 2003. "Syndemics and Public Health: Reconceptualizing Disease in Bio-Social Context." *Medical Anthropology Quarterly* 17 (4): 423–41.

Smith, Neil. 2006. "There's No Such Thing as a Natural Disaster." *Understanding Katrina: Perspectives from the Social Sciences*. http://understandingkatrina.ssrc.org/Smith/.

Sollom, Richard, Chris Beyrer, David Sanders, A. Frank Donaghue, Helen Potts, John Bradshaw, Susannah M Sirkin, Paul Caruso and Gurukarm Khalsa. 2009. "Health in Ruins: A Man-Made Disaster in Zimbabwe." An Emergency Report by Physicians for Human Rights. Washington, DC.

Stellmach, Darryl. 2016. "Coordination in Crisis: The Practice of Medical Humanitarian Emergency." Unpublished DPhil Thesis, University of Oxford.

Stephenson, J. 2009. "Cholera in Zimbabwe." *JAMA: The Journal of the American Medical Association* 301 (3): 263.

Stewart, Frances, and Graham Brown. 2009. "Fragile States." CRISE Working Paper No. 51.

Street, Alice. 2014. "Rethinking Infrastructures for Global Health: A View from West Africa and Papua New Guinea." *Somatosphere*. http://somatosphere.net/?p=9591.

Swanson, M W. 1977. "The Sanitation Syndrome: Bubonic Plague and Urban Native Policy in the Cape Colony, 1900-1909." *Journal of African History* 18 (3): 387–410.

Taylor, Andrew. 2013. *State Failure*. Basingstoke: Palgrave Macmillan.

Tendi, Blessing-Miles. 2010. *Making History in Mugabe's Zimbabwe: Politics, Intellectuals and the Media*. Oxford: Verlag Peter Lang.

2013. "Ideology, Civilian Authority and the Zimbabwean Military." *Journal of Southern African Studies* 39 (4): 829–43.

2014. "The Origins and Functions of Demonisation Discourses in Britain–Zimbabwe Relations (2000–)." *Journal of Southern African Studies* 40 (6): 1–19.

Tibaijuka, Anna Kajumulo. 2005. "Report of the Fact-Finding Mission to Zimbabwe to Assess the Scope and Impact of Operation Murambatsvina." *UN Habitat*.

Ticktin, Miriam. 2011. *Casualties of Care: Immigration and the Politics of Humanitarianism in France*. Berkeley: University of California Press.

Todd, Charles, Sunanda Ray, Farai Madzimbamuto and David Sanders. 2009. "What Is the Way Forward for Health in Zimbabwe?" *The Lancet* 6736 (9): 7–10.

Tomlinson, Roy W., and Peter Wurzel. 1977. "Aspects of Site and Situation." In *Salisbury: A Geographical Survey of the Capital of Rhodesia*, edited by George Kay and Michael Smout, 1–13. London: Hodder & Stoughton.

UNAIDS/WHO. 2000. "Zimbabwe Epidemiological Fact Sheet." New York & Geneva.

Vaughan, Megan. 1991. *Curing Their Ills: Colonial Power and African Illness*. Cambridge: Polity Press.

Venugopal, Rajesh, and Sameer Yasir. 2017. "The Politics of Natural Disasters in Protracted Conflict: The 2014 Flood in Kashmir." *Oxford Development Studies* 45(4): 424–42.

Verheul, Susanne. 2013. "'Rebels' and 'Good Boys': Patronage, Intimidation and Resistance in Zimbabwe's Attorney General's Office after 2000." *Journal of Southern African Studies* 39 (4): 765–82.

Verhoeven, Harry. 2011. "Climate Change, Conflict and Development in Sudan: Global Neo-Malthusian Narratives and Local Power Struggles." *Development and Change* 42 (3): 679–707.

2015. *Water, Civilisation and Power in Sudan: The Political Economy of Military-Islamist State Building*. New York: Cambridge University Press.

Welsh, Marc. 2014. "Resilience and Responsibility: Governing Uncertainty in a Complex World." *Geographical Journal* 180 (1): 15–26.

Werbner, Richard P. 1991. *Tears of the Dead: The Social Biography of an African Family*. Edinburgh: Edinburgh University Press.

White, Luise. 2000. "Telling More: Lies, Secrets, and History." *History and Theory* 39 (4): 11–22.

Whiteside, Alan, and Tony Barnett. 2002. *AIDS in the Twenty-First Century: Disease and Globalization*. Basingstoke: Palgrave Macmillan.

Williams, Gavin. 2003. "Studying Development and Explaining Policies." *Oxford Development Studies* 31 (1): 37–58.

World Bank. 1992. "Zimbabwe: Financing Health Services." Washington, DC.

World Health Organization. 2006. "Cholera Country Profile: Mozambique." *Global Task Force on Cholera Control*. www.who.int/cholera/countries/Mozambique country profile.pdf.

2009. "Cholera in Zimbabwe – Update 2." *Global Alert and Response*. www.who.int/csr/don/2009_02_20/en/.

World Health Organization/Government of Zimbabwe: Ministry of Health. 2011. "Intersectoral Actions in Response to Cholera in Zimbabwe: From Emergency Response to Institution Building." In *World*

Conference on Social Determinants of Health. Rio De Janeiro. www.who.int/sdhconference.

2013. "Zimbabwe Cholera Outbreak Response 2008–2013." Joint Cholera Initiative for Southern Africa. Johannesburg.

Yamba, C. Bawa. 1997. "Cosmologies in Turmoil: Witchfinding and AIDS in Chiawa, Zambia." *Africa: Journal of the International African Institute* 67 (2): 200–23.

Yoshikuni, Tsuneo. 2007. *African Urban Experiences in Colonial Zimbabwe: A Social History of Harare before 1925*. Harare: Weaver Press.

Youde, J. 2010. "Don't Drink the Water: Politics and Cholera in Zimbabwe." *International Journal: Canada's Journal of Global Policy Analysis* 65 (3): 687–704.

Young, Allan. 1982. "The Anthropologies of Illness and Sickness." *Annual Review of Anthropology* 11: 257–85.

Zartman, William. 1995. *Collapsed States: The Disintegration and Restoration of Legitimate Authority*. Boulder: Lynne Rienner Publishers.

Zimbabwe Association of Doctors for Human Rights. 2009. "Cholera in a Time of Health System Collapse: Violations of Health Rights and the Cholera Outbreak." Harare.

Zimbabwe Coalition on Debt and Development. 2013. "Towards a Pro-People Framework in Water Management: An Assessment of the Political-Economy of Water Service Delivery in Harare." Harare. www.zimcodd.org/sites/default/files/research/Harare Water Research.pdf.

Zimbabwe Government. 1981. "Growth with Equity: An Economic Policy Statement." Harare.

Zimbabwe Lawyers for Human Rights. 2008. "ZLHR Holds Government Accountable for Avoidable Cholera Deaths." *Kubatana*. http://archive.kubatana.net/html/archive/hr/080925zlhr.asp?sector=health&year=2008&range_start=61.

ZINWA. 2011. "About Us." *Zimbabwe National Water Authority*. www.zinwa.co.zw/about-us/.

Index